Professional Men's Hairdressing

THE ART OF CUTTING AND STYLING

Guy Kremer and Jacki Wadeson

PHOTOGRAPHY: BARRY COOK

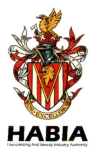

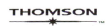 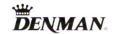 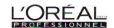 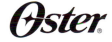

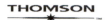

For more information, contact Thomson, High Holborn House, 50–51 Bedford Row, London WC1R 4LR or visit us on the World Wide Web at:
http://www.thomsonlearning.co.uk

British Library Cataloguing-in-Publication Data
A catalogue record for this book is available from the British Library

ISBN 1-86152-902-3

Photographs on chapter openers © Marc Atkins
Designed and typeset by LewisHallam

Printed in Italy by G. Canale & C.

Contents

Acknowledgements

Hair: Guy Kremer
Assisted by: Charlie Manns and Guillaume Vappereau
Colour: L'Oréal Professionnel
Brushes and combs: Denman International Ltd
Clippers: Oster Professional Products GmbH.
Backwash and hair care: L'Oréal Professionnel
Styling products: L'Oréal Professionnel tecni.art
Clothes styling: Mark O'Connor and James Thomas
Photography: Barry Cook
Editor: Jacki Wadeson

With special thanks to:
Alan Richardson, Mai-Britt Rasmussen, Gaynor Hodge, Catherine McMahon, Jane McCarthy,
Kay Connelly, Marie Audemard and Carole Le Roux of L'Oréal Professionnel,
Jonathan S. King, Maria Stafford and Lisa Stewart, Denman,
Alex Queralt, Oster Professional Products GmbH.

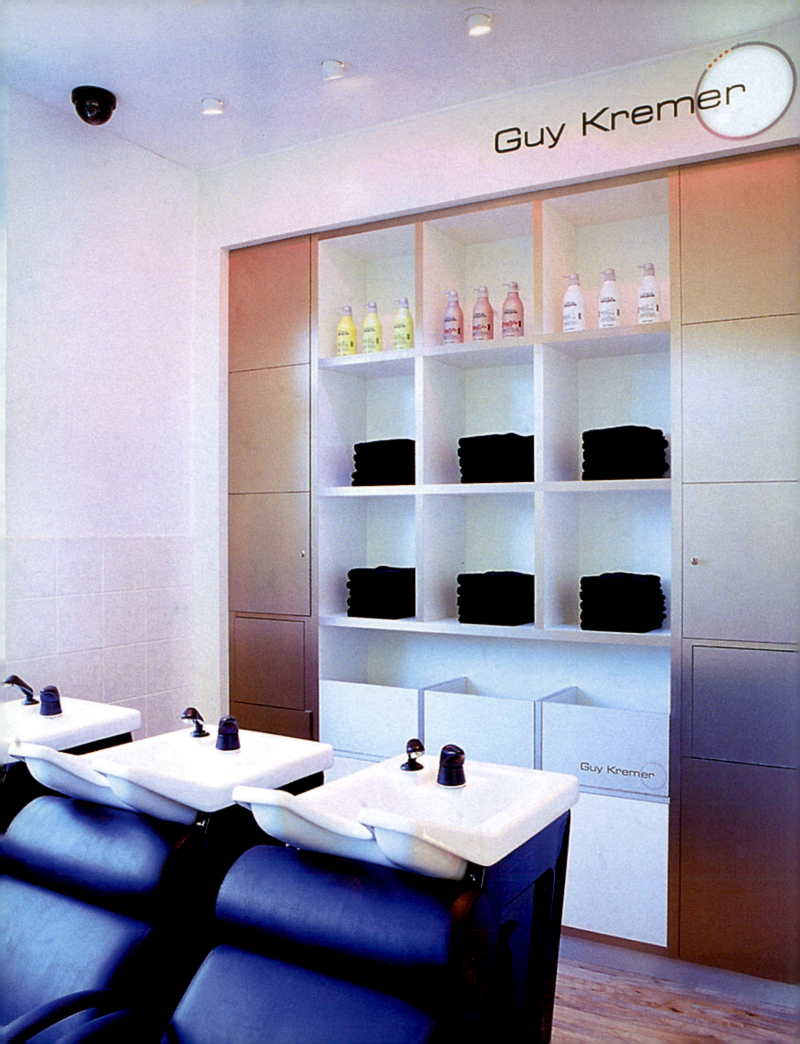

Introduction

Guy Kremer is internationally renowned and sought after worldwide for his cutting and styling expertise. Voted as Fellowship Hairdresser of the Year (1997), named as one the World's Top 75 Educators of the century by USA industry bible, Modern Salon, (1999); winner of the AIPP Men's Award (2000) and his salon was the first to win the coveted L'Oréal Colour Trophy Men's Image Award (1998).

Winner of the Southern Stylist of the Year, for three years in succession, 1988; 1989 and 1990 he is a member of the British Hairdressing Awards Hall of Fame. In 1995 and 2001 his salon won the L'Oréal Colour Trophy – a coup in the world of hairdressing.

Keen to motivate and inspire others Guy is in great demand for seminars and shows. He believes in sharing his artistry and experience with other hairdressers and has the uncanny knack of combining the classic with the funky to create inspirational yet commercial men's hairdressing.

In this book, Guy shows, step-by-step, how to create 25 cutting edge looks using a combination of clipper, scissor and razor cutting techniques. The full colour style gallery offers a further choice of 25 inspirational styles.

When not travelling the world, conducting shows and seminars, Guy is based at his state-of-the art salon in Winchester, a L'Oréal Professional approved colour expert salon. Celebrities, models and movie stars including Graham Souness, Roger Waters and John Sopel as well as designers, Isabell Kristensen and Maria Grachvogel are amongst his clientele.

Jacki Wadeson

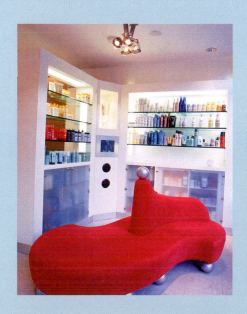
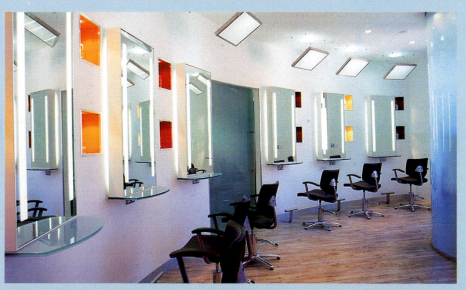

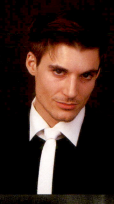

Ska

COLLECTION

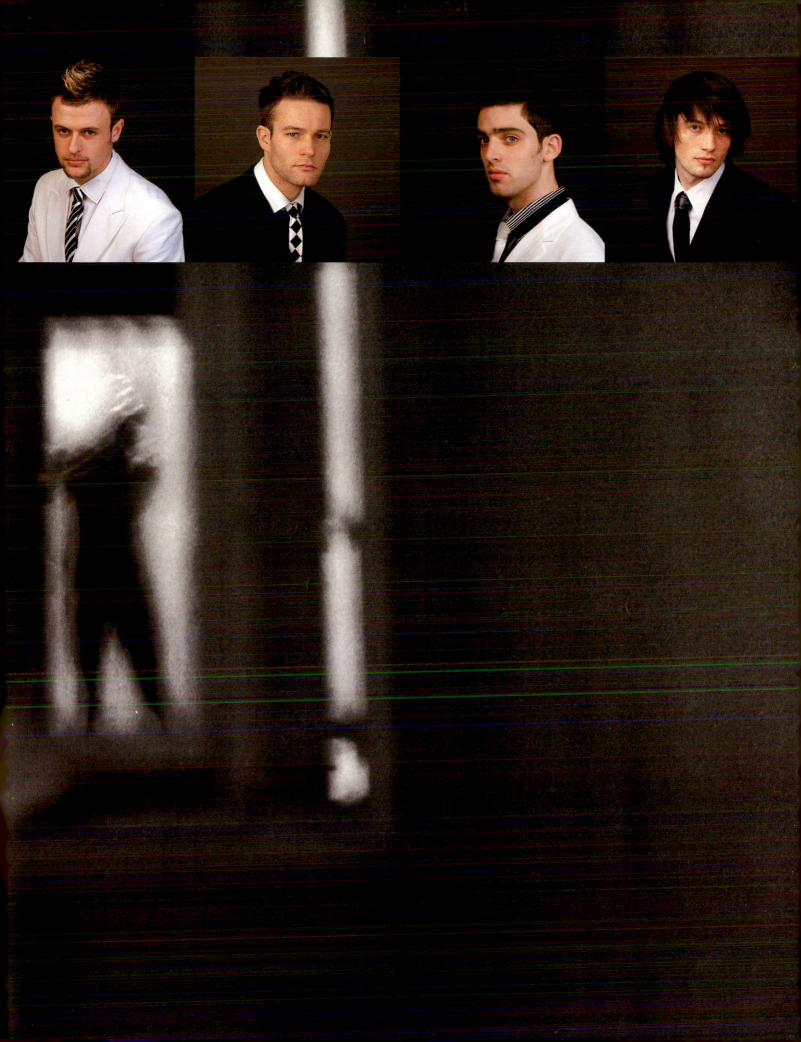

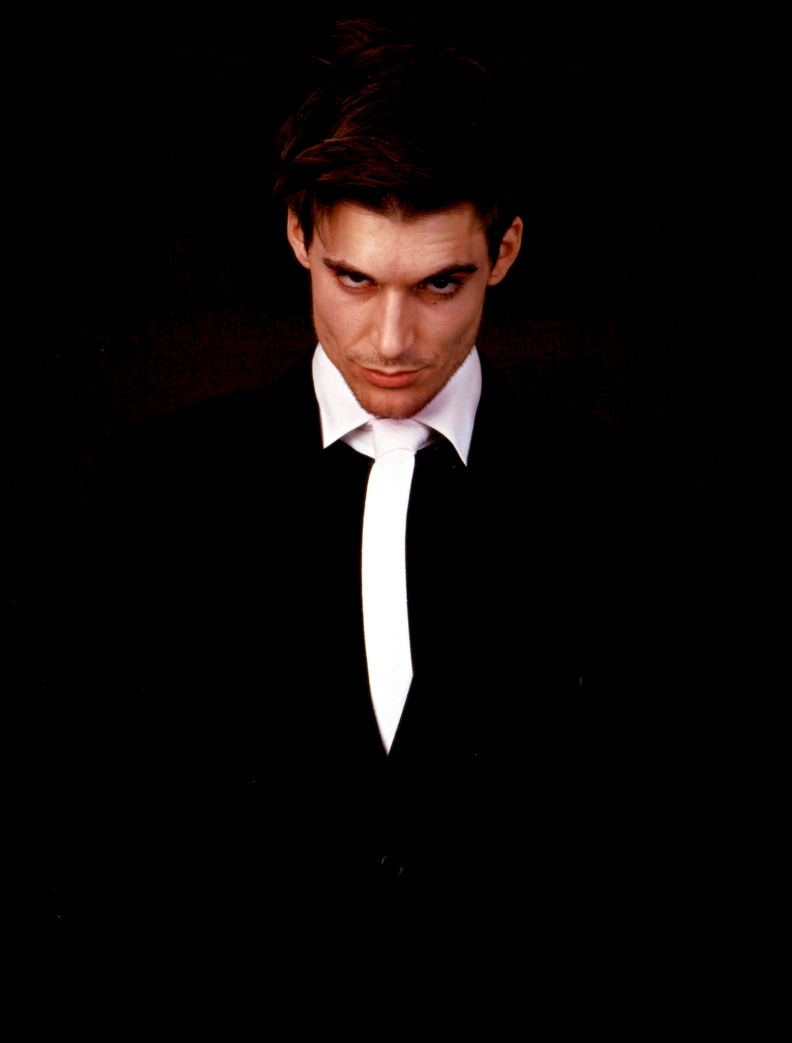

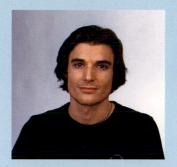

TOBY

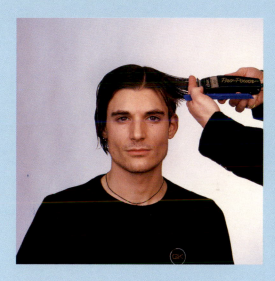

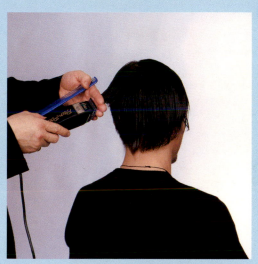

From a side parting, elevate first section to 45 degrees and use clipper to remove bulk of hair.

Working above occipital bone elevate hair to 45 degrees to give guideline and remove bulk of hair.

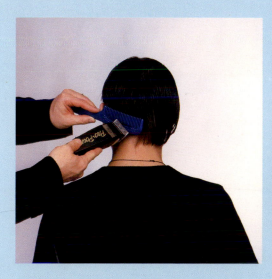

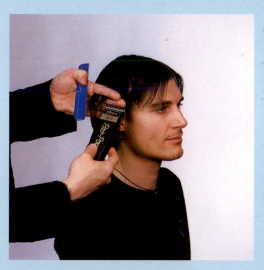

Work clipper over comb from neckline to occipital bone throughout back section.

Proceed to side section, elevating hair to 45 degrees and removing bulk up to the guideline.

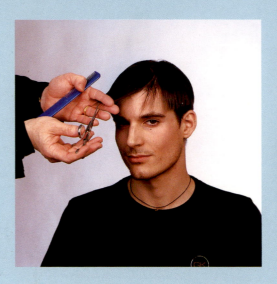

Point cut fringe section to remove length and to texturise.

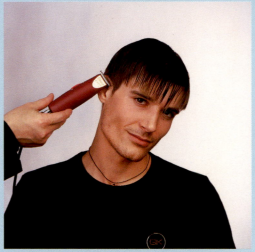

Use finisher clipper to tidy hairline round front and back of ears.

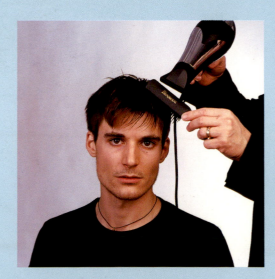

Apply tecni.art Volume + mousse for volume and control, before blow-drying with a Classic Styling Brush.

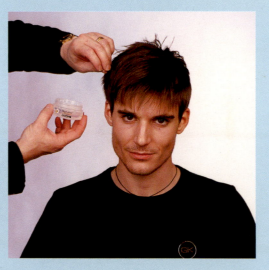

Use fingers to apply tecni.art Digit gloss to hair to accentuate texture and add gloss.

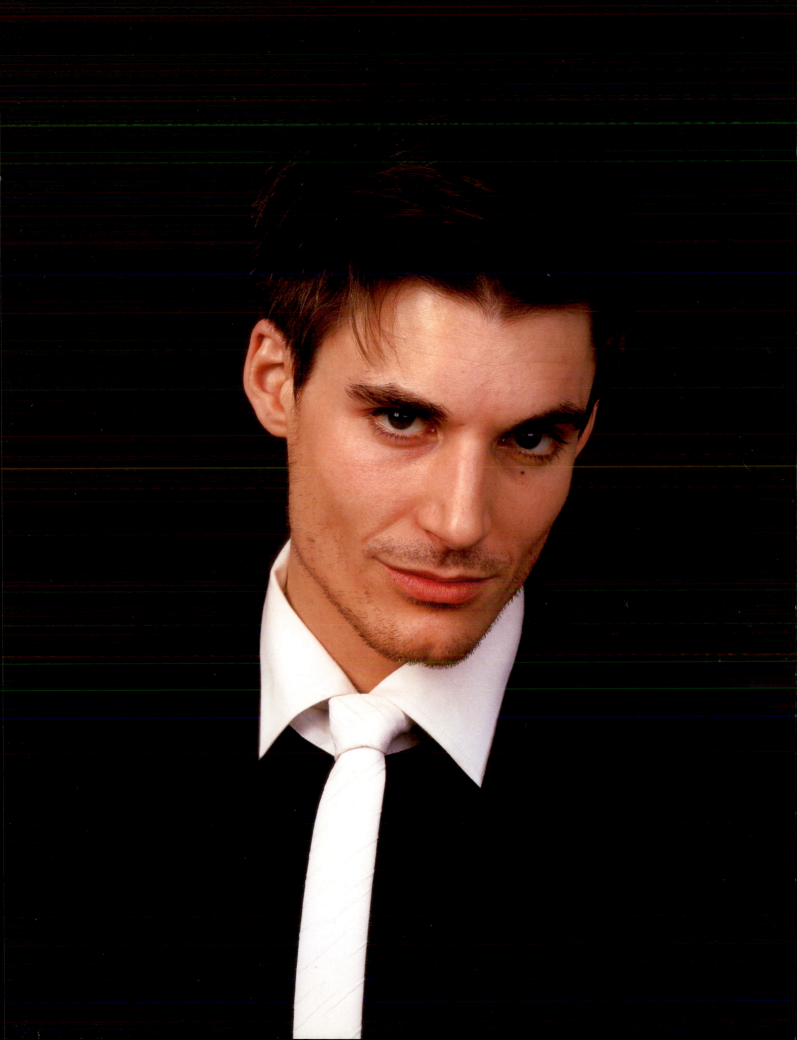

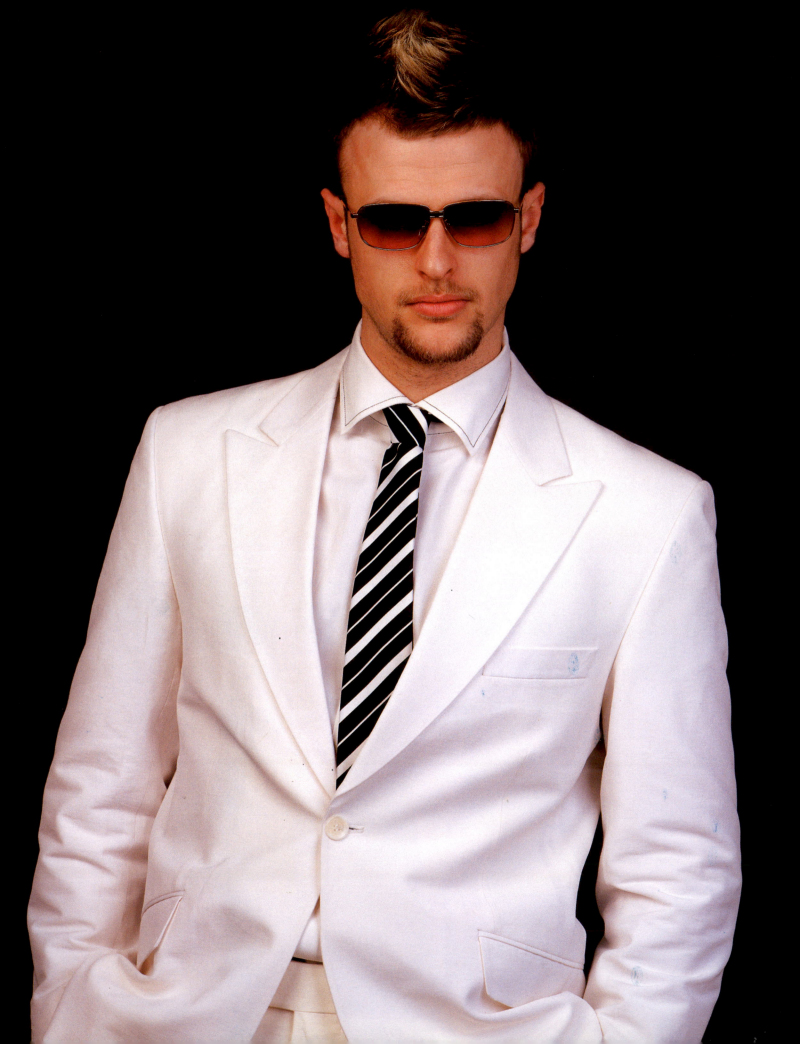

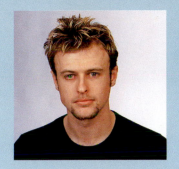

PAUL

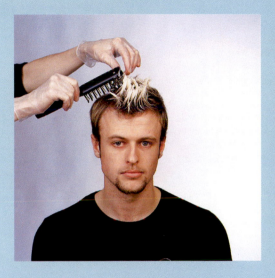

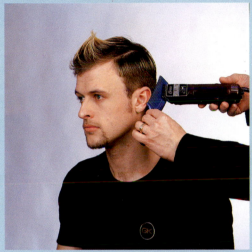

Blow-dry hair upwards then use a Tunnel Vent brush to apply Platine Precision pre-lightening powder (1 scoop + 45 ml of 30 vol (9%) L'Oréal Professionnel cream oxidant) to central section. Leave to process then rinse before shampooing.

Using clipper over comb work up from neckline to ear level.

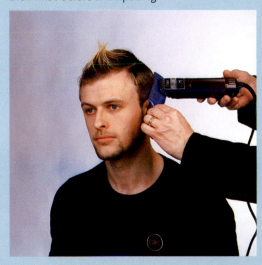

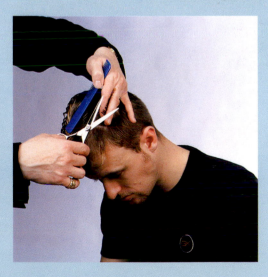

Continue from ear level to temple in same manner. Work back and other side section in same way.

Take a horizontal section on crown and remove length by cutting straight.

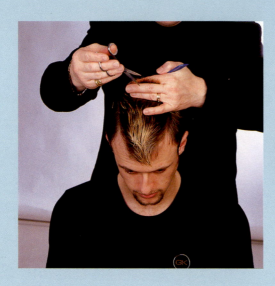

Take a square section on crown, comb upwards and chip into ends.

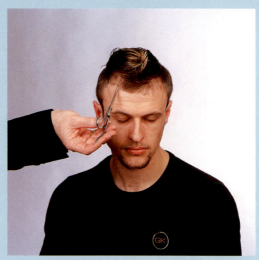

Strengthen front hairline by point cutting into it so hair is left quite short.

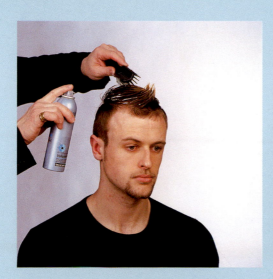

Use a Vent Brush to distribute tecni.art Volume + mousse through hair.

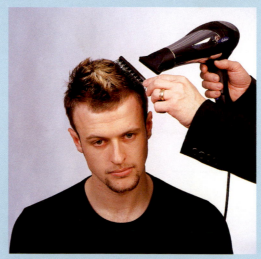

Dry using a nozzle attachment and directing heat upwards to create quiff.

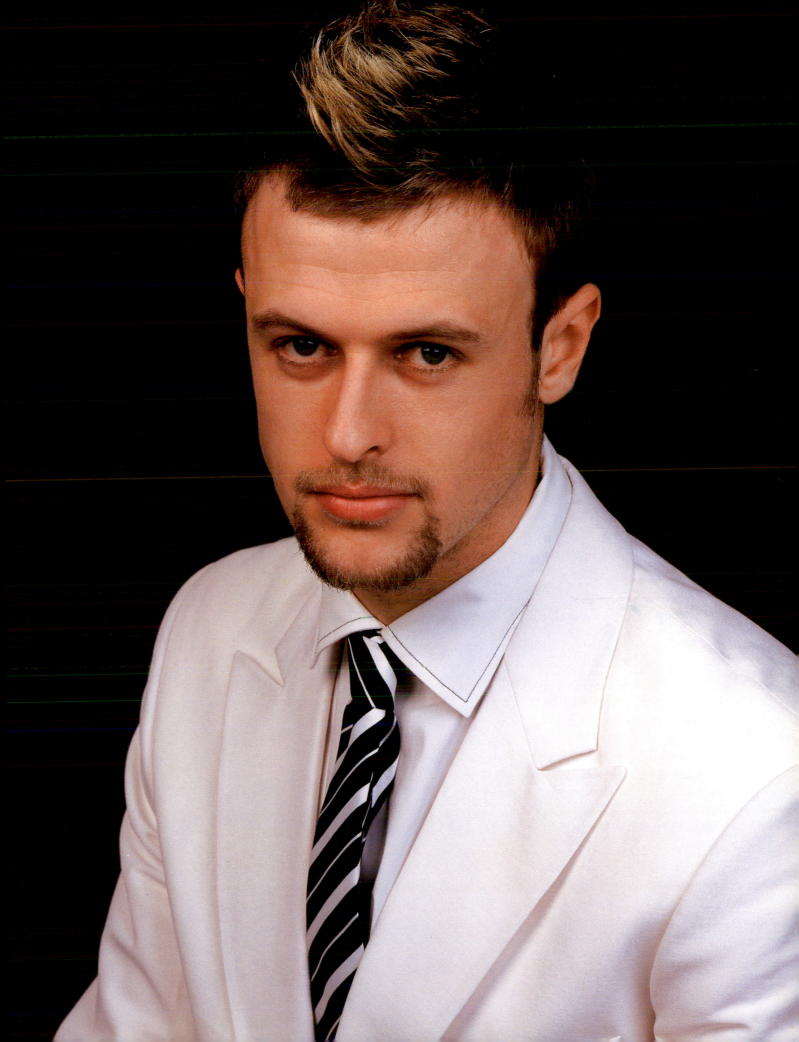

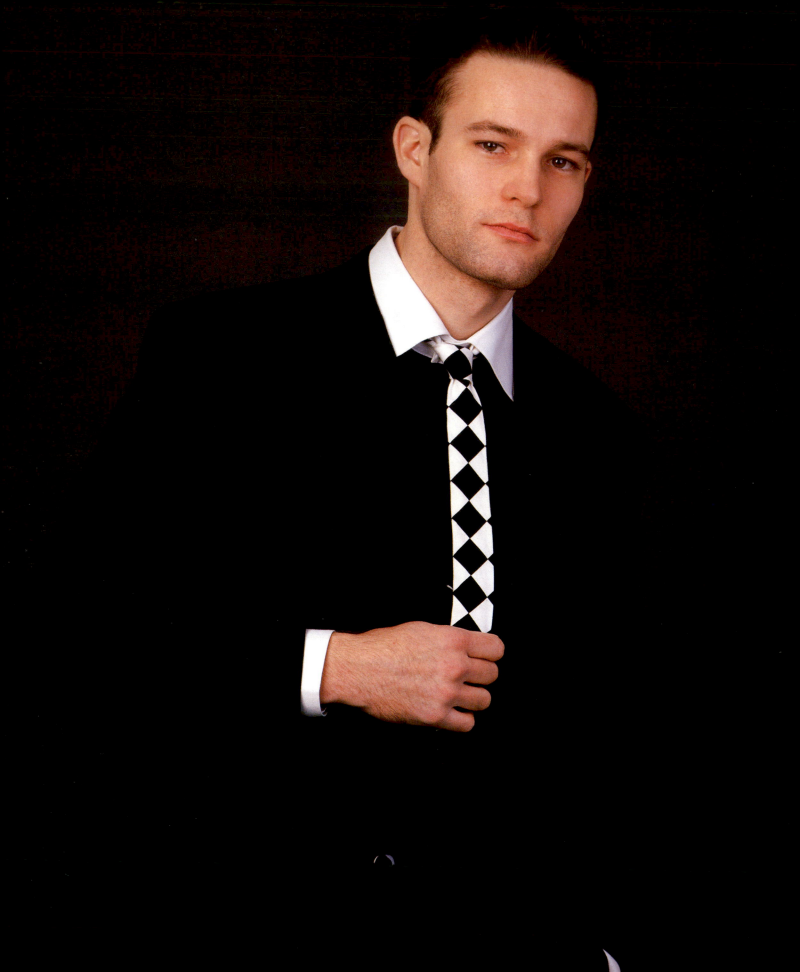

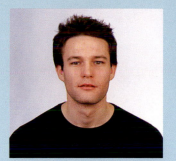

GARETH

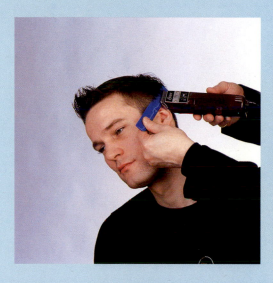

Use clipper over comb to cut side hair working around perimeter to give a short finish.

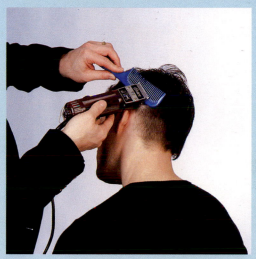

Working with clipper over comb to give more elevation to graduation, work from above the ear.

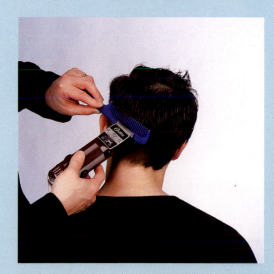

Clipper back using a comb to lift hair whilst moving clippers upwards. The base of the comb is pressed against the scalp to maintain control.

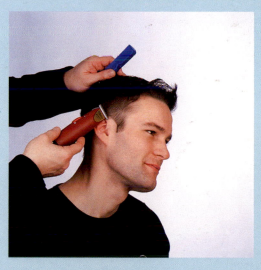

Use finisher clipper to clean perimeter round ear.

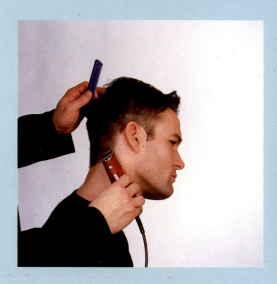

Use finisher clipper to clean neckline.

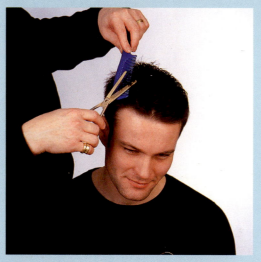

Create texture at the crown using a comb and thinning scissors to remove weight and length.

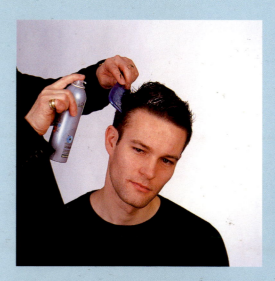

Use a comb to distribute tecni.art Volume Lift Directional mousse from roots to ends of hair.

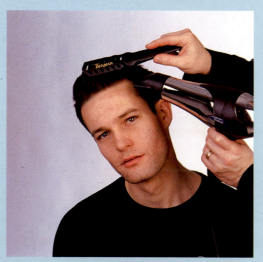

Dry with a Vent Brush and nozzle attachment on the dryer to achieve further root lift.

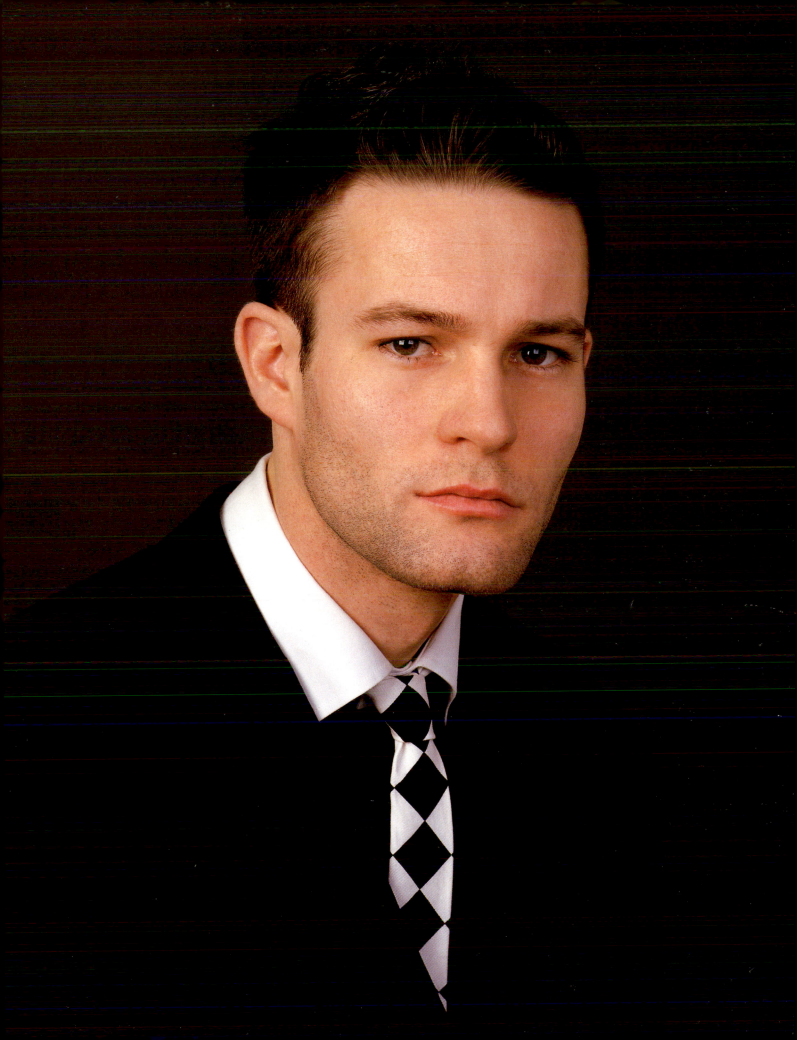

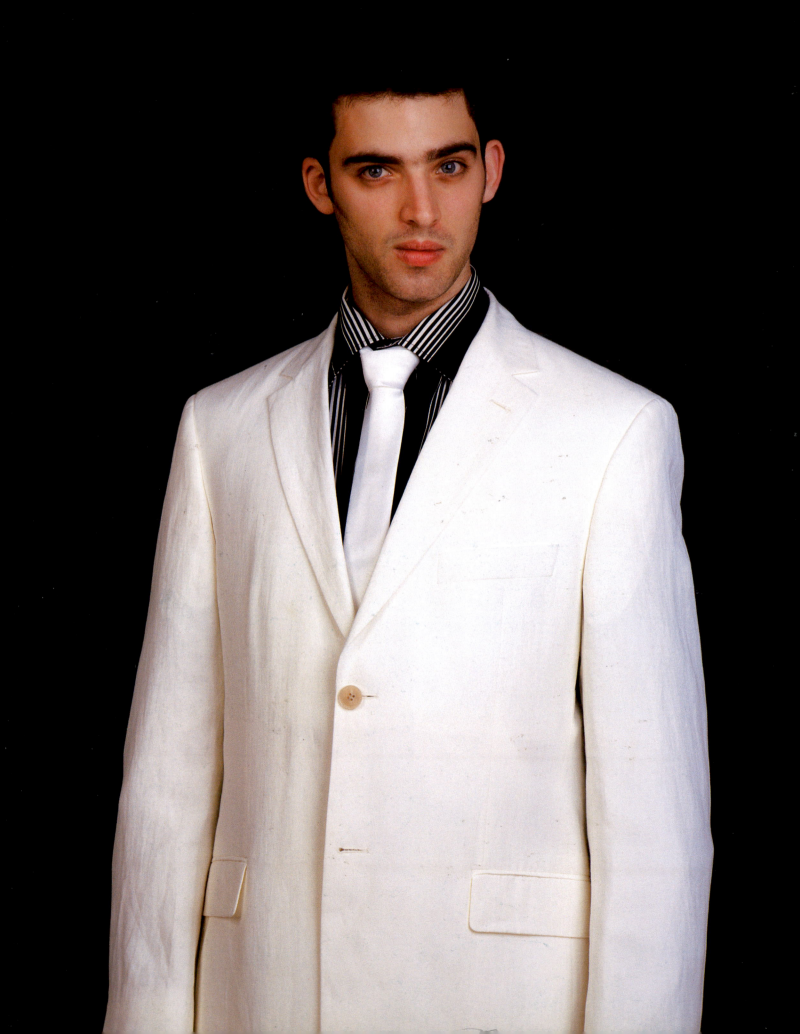

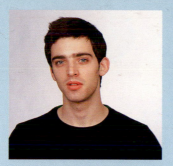

JOSE

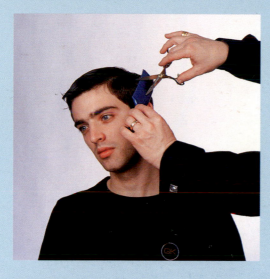

Make a side parting and use scissor over comb to remove length and create texture at side.

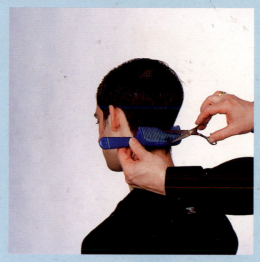

Again use scissor over comb to cut back section from nape area to occipital bone.

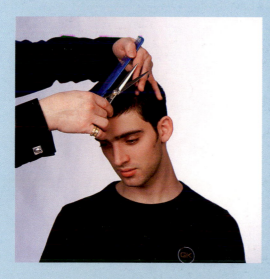

Take vertical sections on front and cut straight.

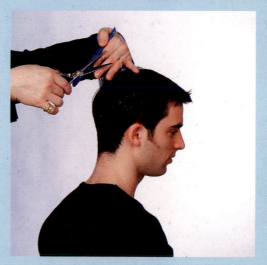

Take vertical sections on crown and cut straight.

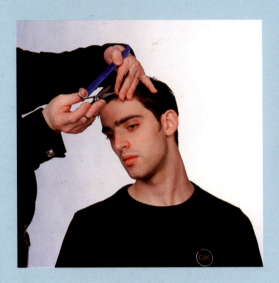

Point cut into front hair to texturise.

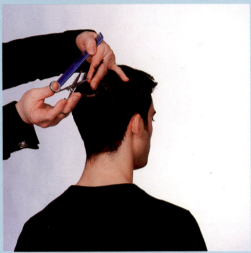

Point cut crown area.

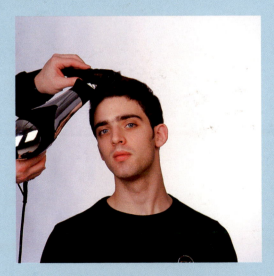

Dry hair using a Tunnel Vent Brush and concentrator attachment on the dryer to get lift.

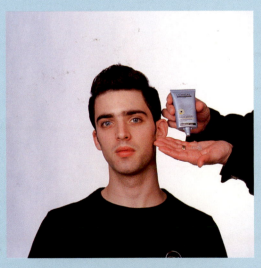

Apply tecni.art Gloss polish to hand then work through the hair to achieve a shiny polished finish.

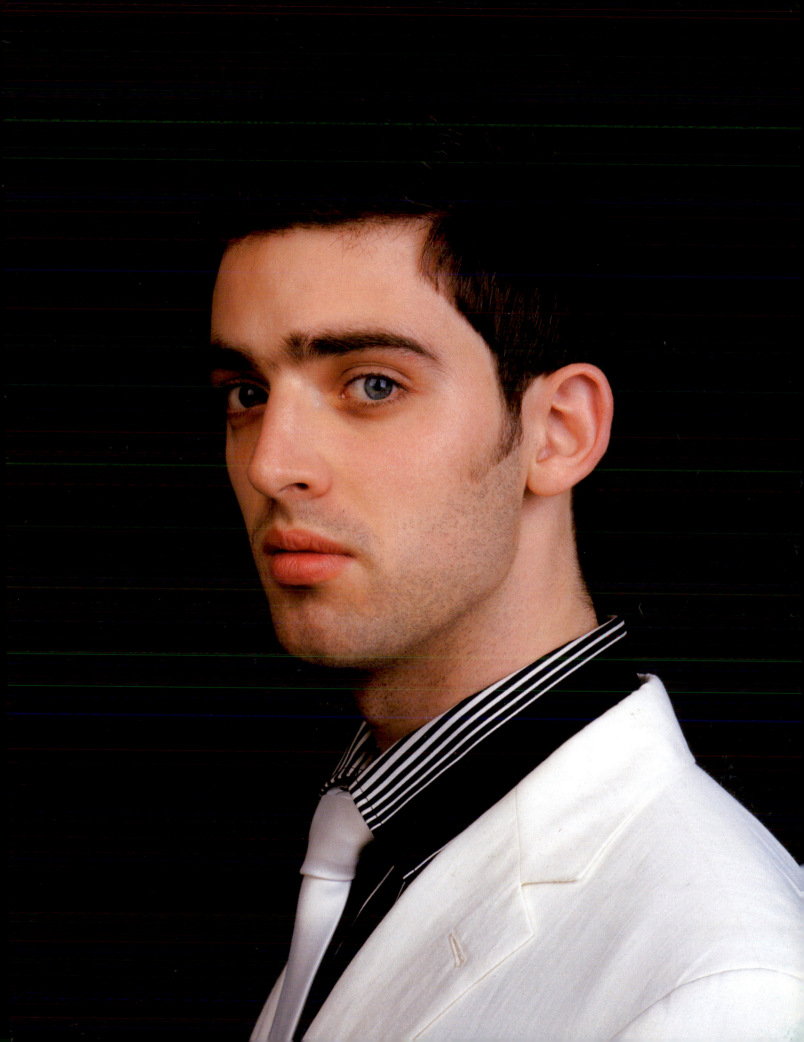

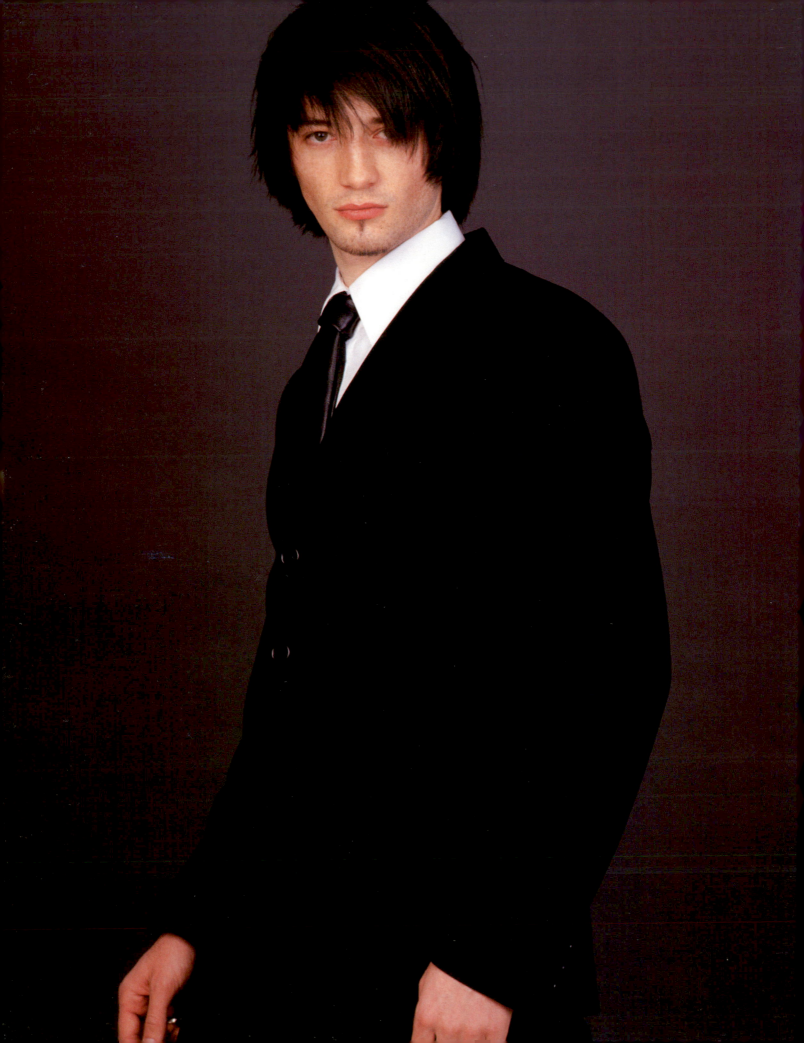

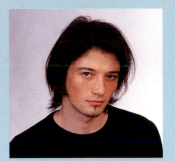

MARIO

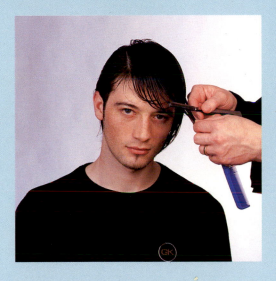

From a side-parting razor cut 4cm of fringe to give texture using feathering movements to remove weight.

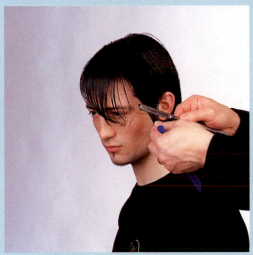

Overdirect the side sections removing weight and length.

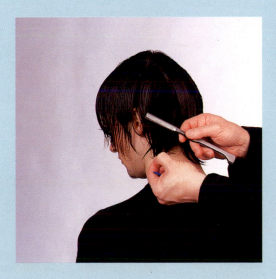

Take an 'orange' segment section at back and over-direct hair to 45 degrees removing weight and length.

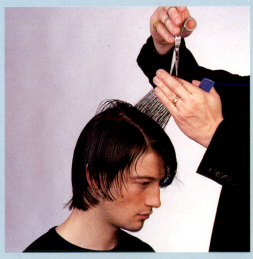

Take a section vertical to the parting and point cut to texturise.

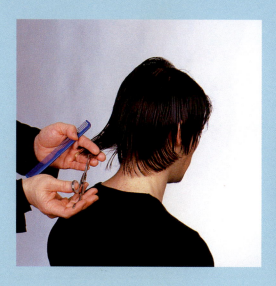

Point cut perimeter.

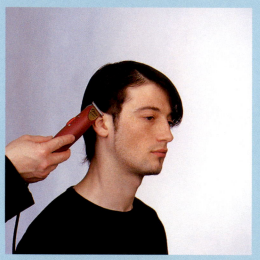

Use finisher clipper to clean round ears.

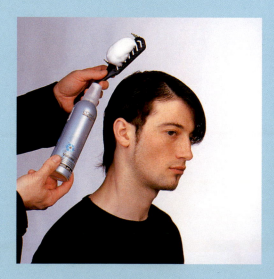

Use tecni.art Volume + mousse, apply to Vent Brush and distribute through hair.

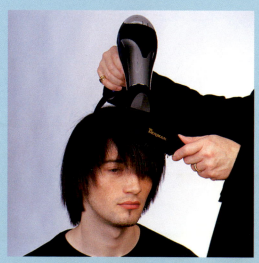

Blow-dry using a nozzle attachment on dryer and a small Paddle Brush.

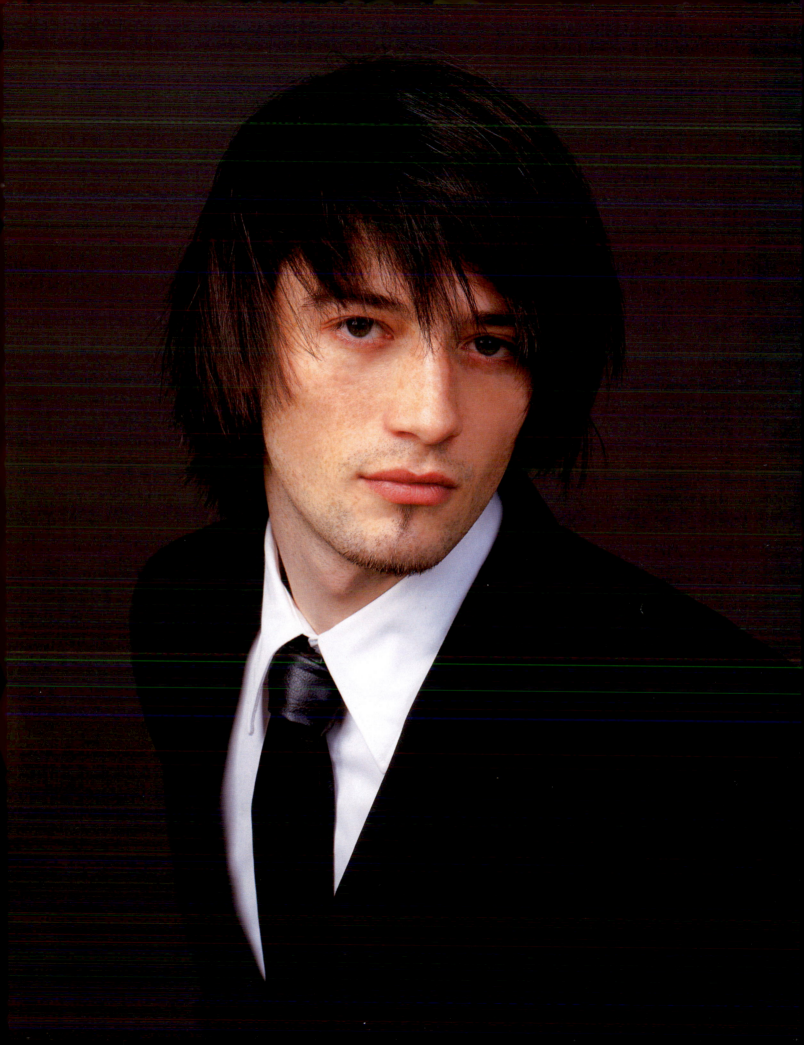

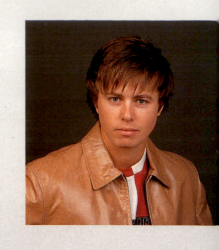

Urban

COLLECTION

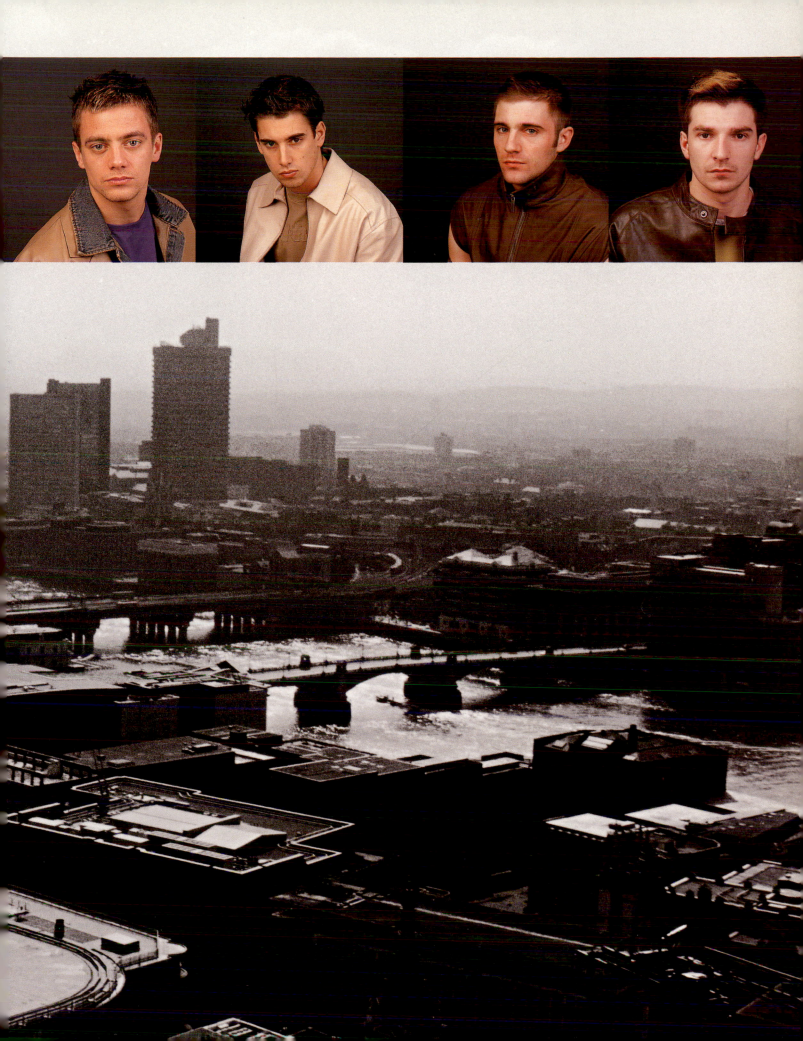

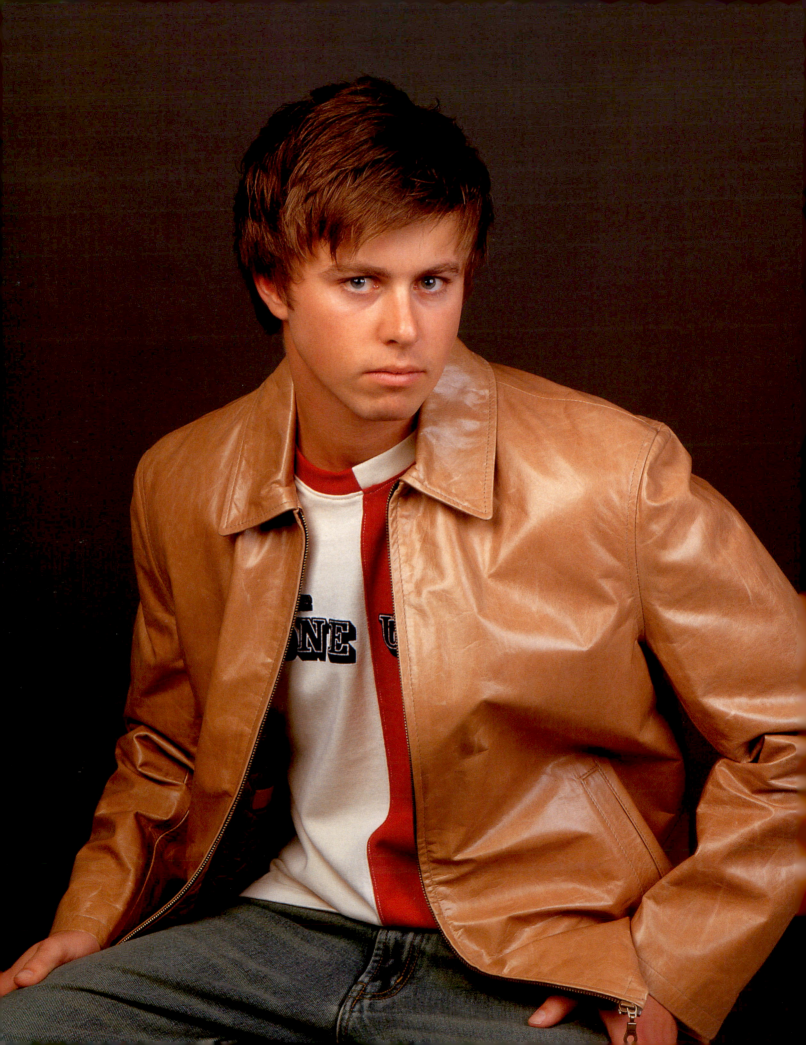

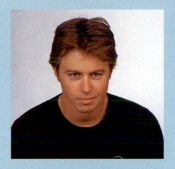

JAMES

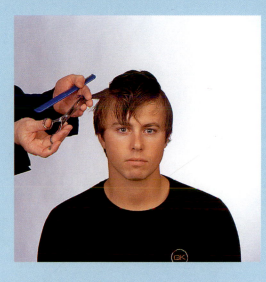

Box section crown hair. Now, take a vertical section from side, elevate to 45 degrees and cut into section using backhand technique.

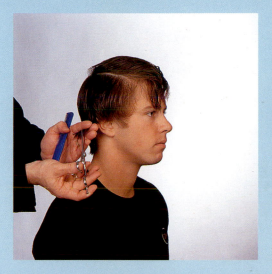

On side, overdirect and cut into section.

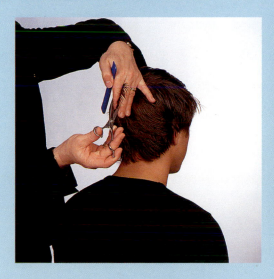

Take a vertical section at the back and cut into it at 1.5cm intervals all the way up.

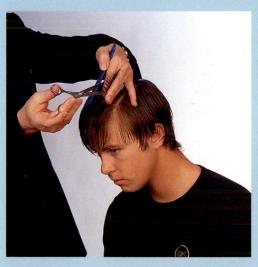

Work on box section at crown, take a vertical elevation and cut into it at 1.5cm intervals all the way along.

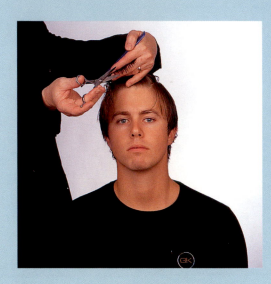

Check box section for balance.

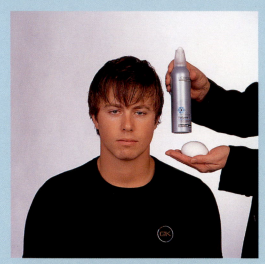

Dispense tecni.art Volume + mousse onto hand then distribute evenly through the hair.

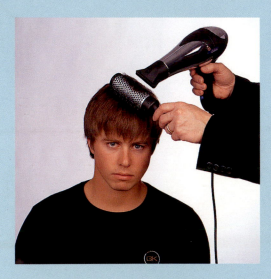

Blow-dry using a Thermo™ Hot Curl Brush and diffuser attachment.

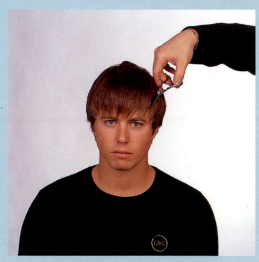

Finish by slice cutting into fringe area.

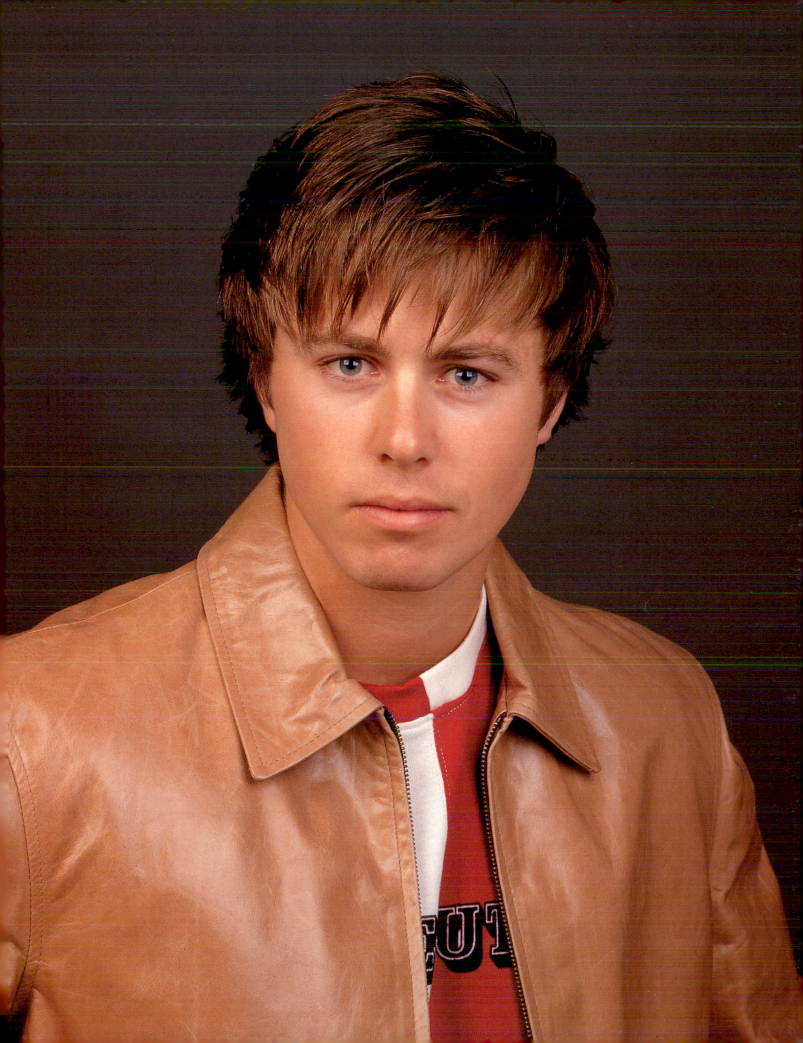

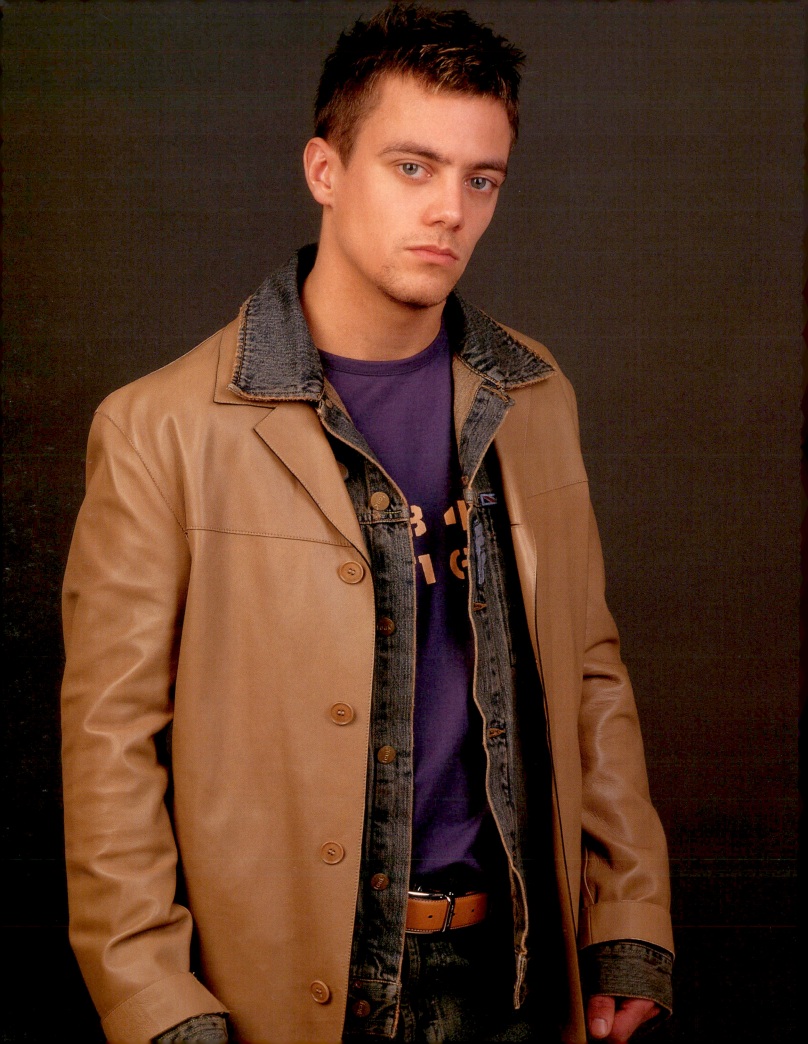

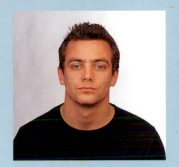

FORBES

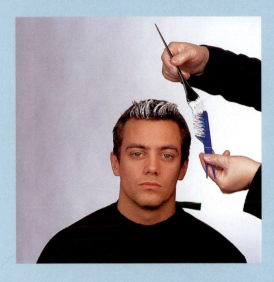

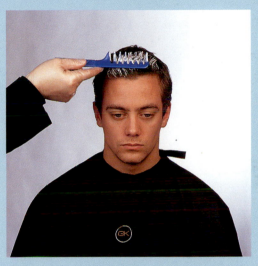

Apply Platine Precision pre-lightening powder (1 scoop + 45ml of 30 vol (9%) L'Oréal Professionnel Cream Oxidant) to comb and apply to front hair.

Continue applying pre-lightner through front section. Leave to process then rinse thoroughly and shampoo.

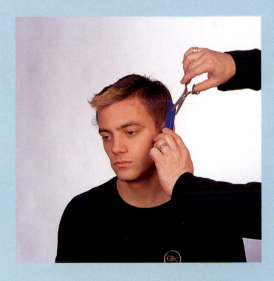

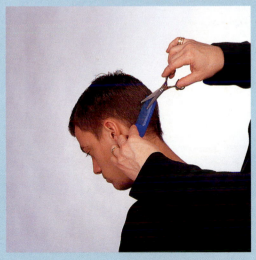

From a side parting use scissor over comb to cut from ear to temple.

Cut the back hair from nape to just above occipital bone again using scissor over comb technique. Proceed through back section in same manner.

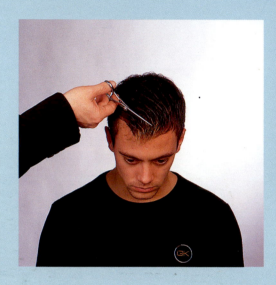

Bias cut crown using diagonal strokes of the scissors.

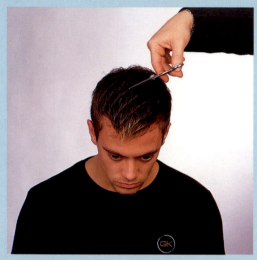

Now bias cut in opposite direction.

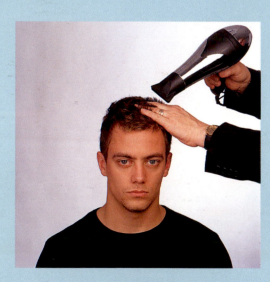

Use fingers to lift and ruffle hair as you dry.

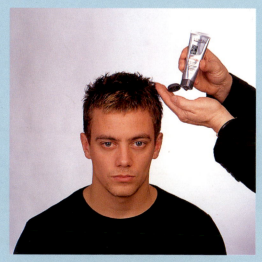

Apply tecni.art Fix boost to palm of hand then work through hair to give hold.

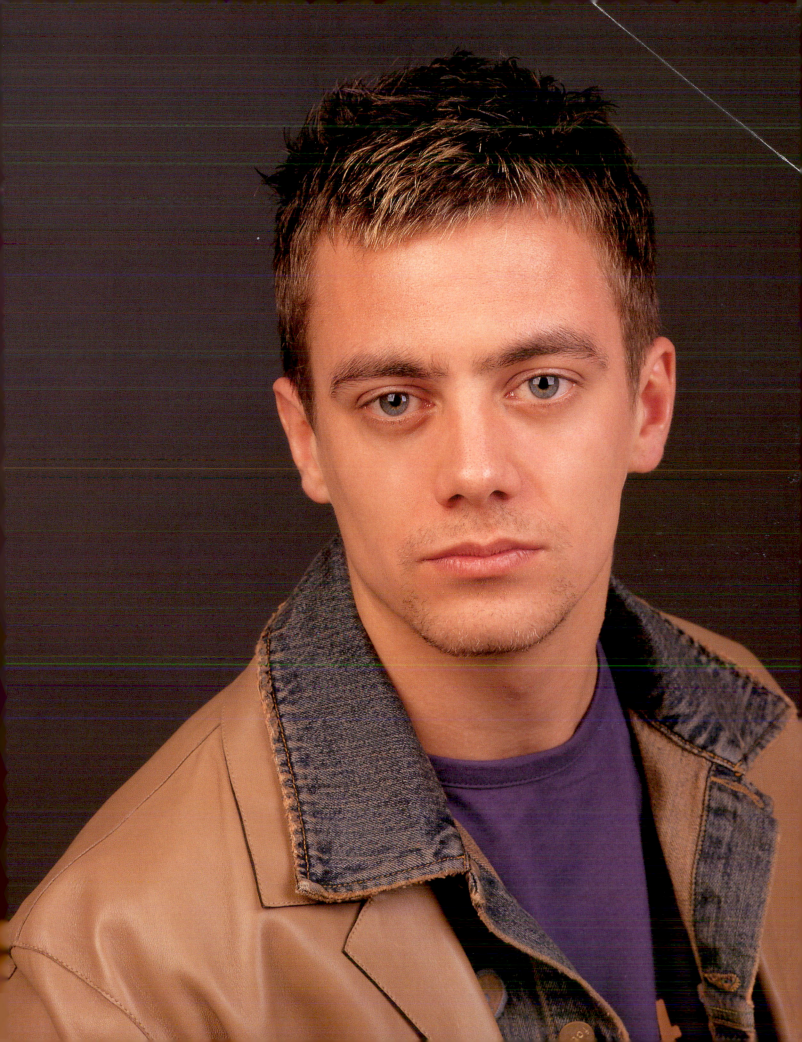

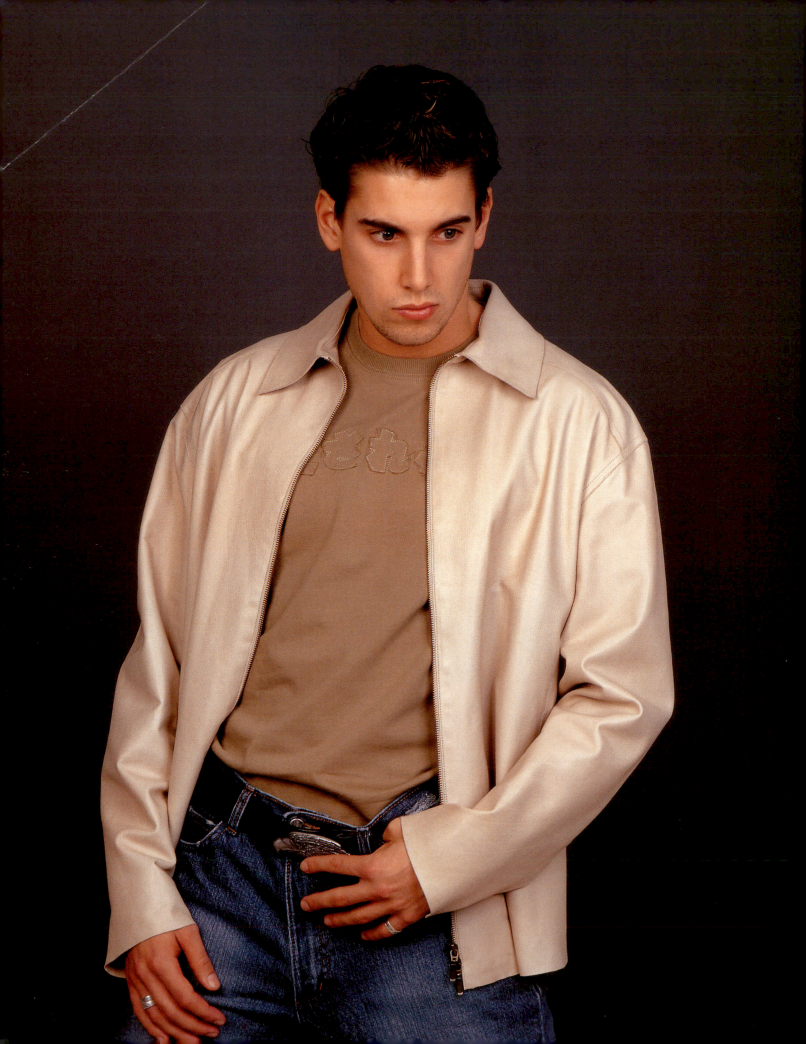

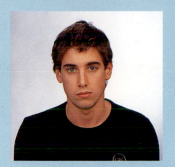

RUSSELL

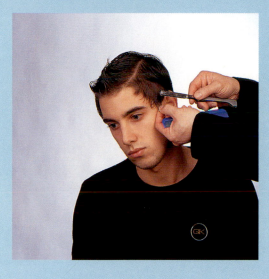

Working from a side parting use a razor to remove length and weight over ear to temple.

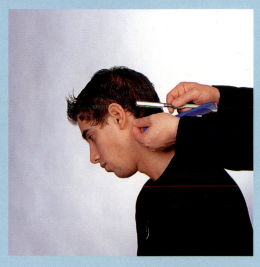

Take vertical sections through back section from crown to nape, continue using razor technique to remove length and weight. Continue through back section in the same manner.

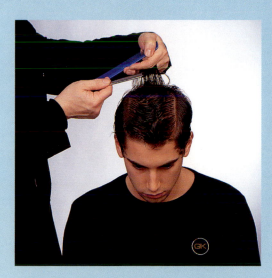

Take horizontal sections on the crown and work with razor in same way.

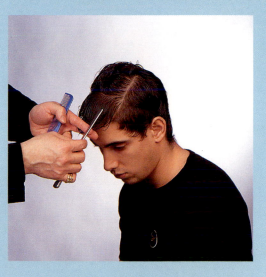

Box section fringe area. Razor using maximum pressure for first stroke and lighter pressure for following strokes thus removing weight and length.

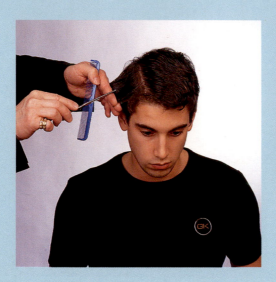

Finish by texturising sides, point cutting with end of the razor.

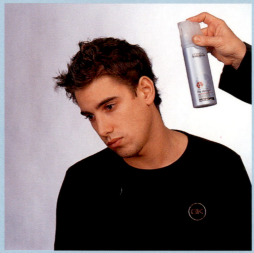

Mist hair with tecni.art Fix design.

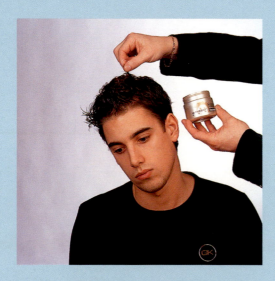

Sculpt sections using tecni.art a-head GUM.

OPEN RAZORS

Open razors are usually used in barbering. They have either a fixed blade, which must be sharpened or set, or a detachable blade, which is disposable. Open razors, also known as 'cut throat' razors, have a hinged handle that closes to protect the blade when not in use.
Open razors are extremely sharp and must be treated with respect. Keep the handle closed to cover the blade when not in use, and especially when carrying or passing the razor. Never place a razor in your pocket. Always keep razors out of reach of any children who may be in the salon. When passing an open razor, the handle must always be closed. In addition, wrap your hand around the closed razor to prevent it from opening accidentally.

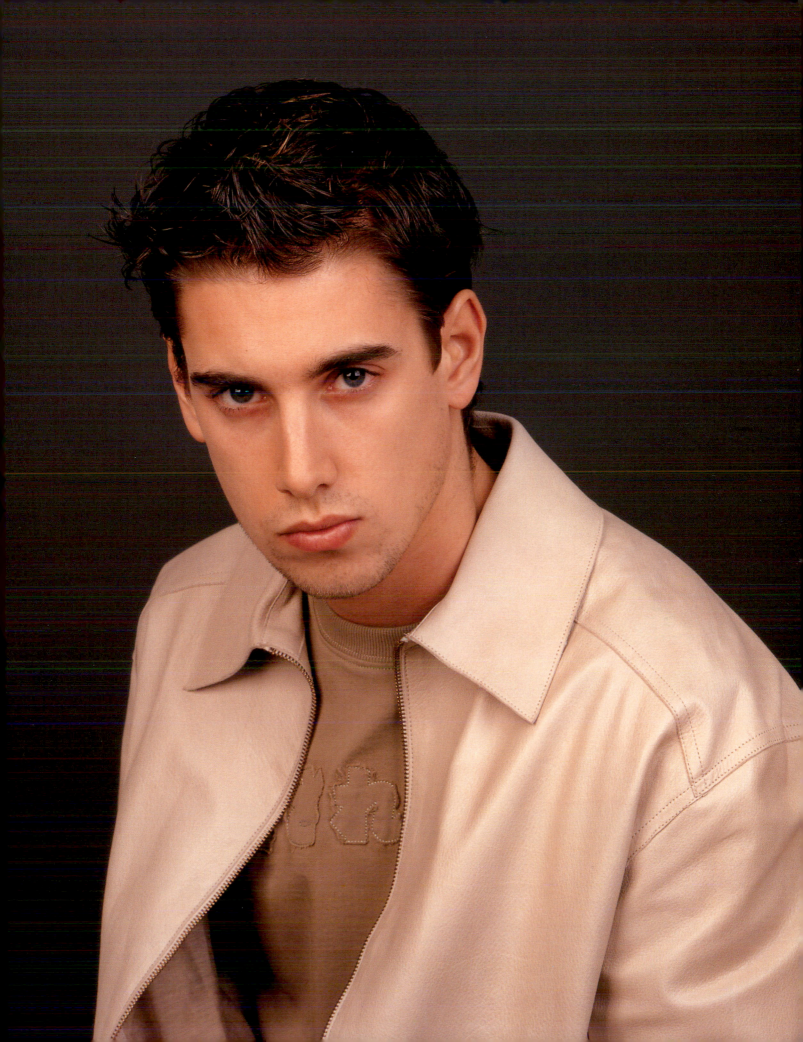

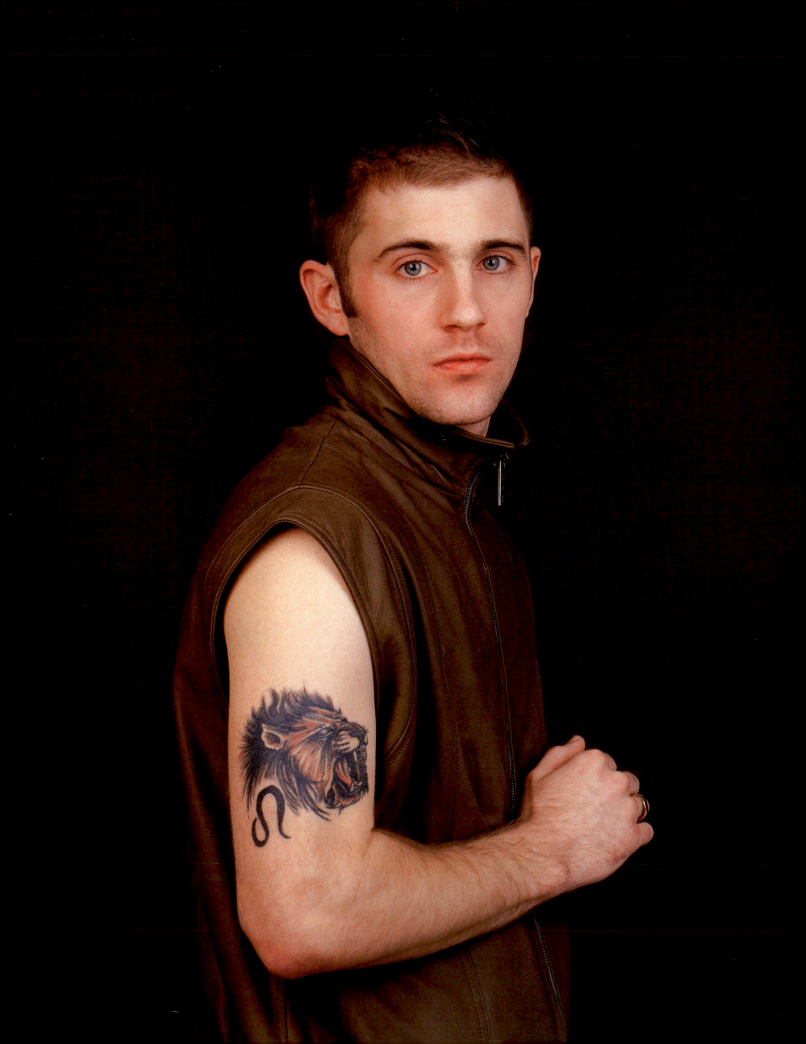

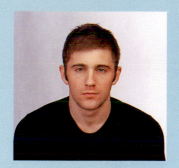

LEE

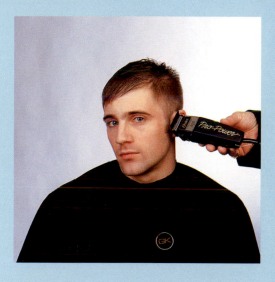

Work on one side using clippers with blending guard to remove hair from sideburns and above ear.

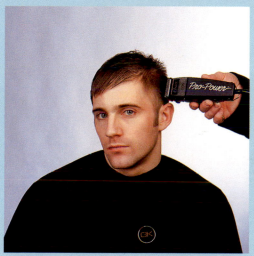

Change to No.2 guard working upwards from above the ear to occipital bone at back and to temple at front.

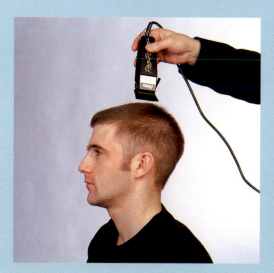

Using the No.4 guard cut crown hair leaving a 2.5cm triangular section at front.

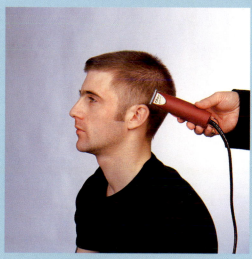

Use finisher clipper round contour of ear.

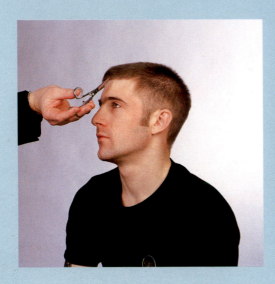

Point cut round the front area to texturise.

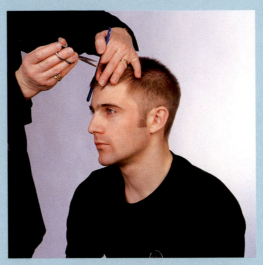

Take vertical sections from front triangle and chip into ends creating more texture.

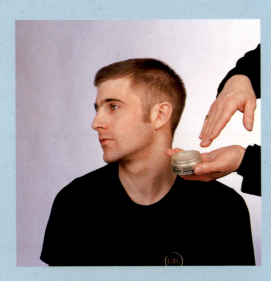

Apply a little tecni.art a-head CLAY into palm of hand and warm with fingers.

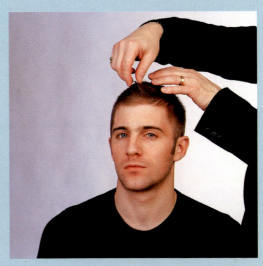

Work tecni.art a-head CLAY through the hair to give a matt textured finish.

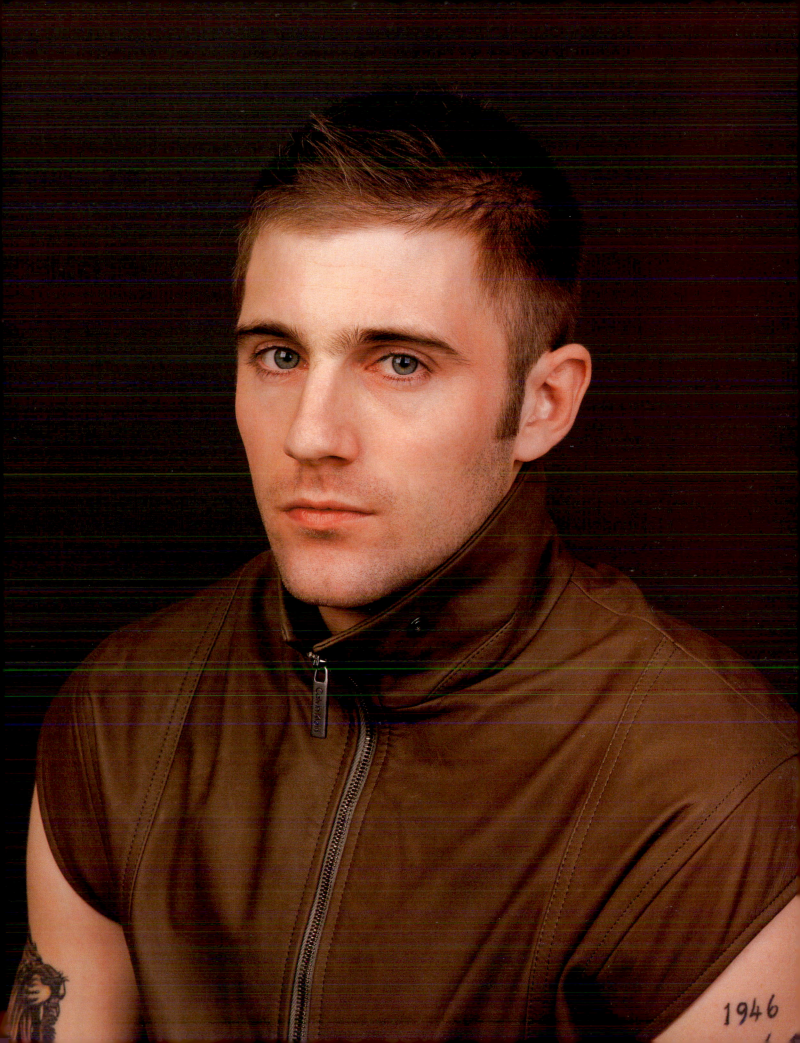

1946

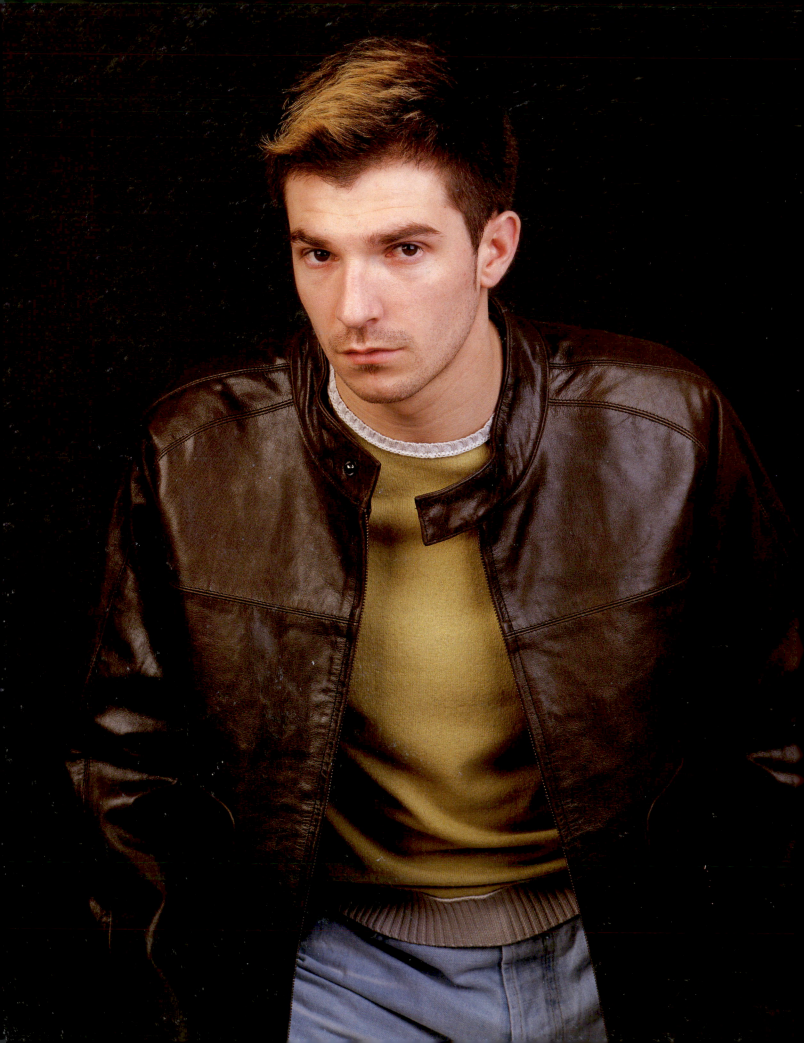

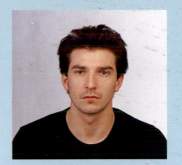

MARK

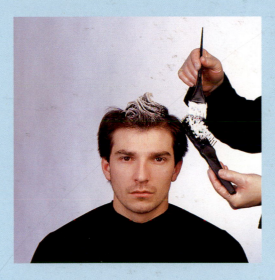

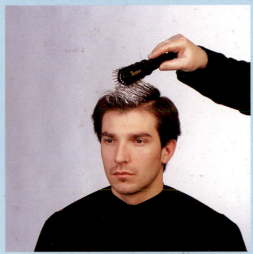

Section off crown hair. Apply Platine Precision pre-lightening powder (1 scoop + 45ml of 30 vol (9%) L'Oréal Professionnel cream oxidant) to Vent Brush, then begin application to hair.

Continue applying Platine Precision distributing with Vent Brush. Leave to process then rinse thoroughly and shampoo.

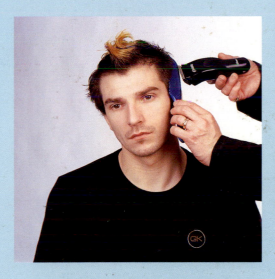

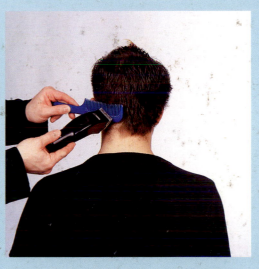

Using clipper over comb, work on first side removing bulk and weight.

Work on back in same manner from nape upwards stopping just above occipital bone. Work other side in same way.

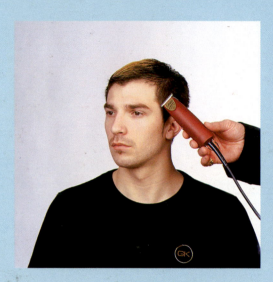

Use finisher clipper to clean hair from around ears.

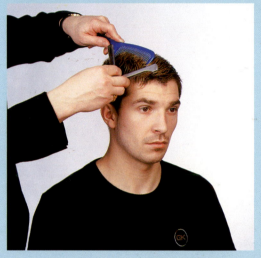

Comb front hair flat then 'lick' hair with razor to gently remove weight and length.

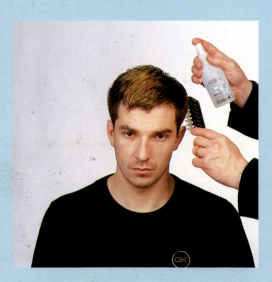

Spray hair with tecni.art airfluid which adds lightness and control to thick and frizzy hair.

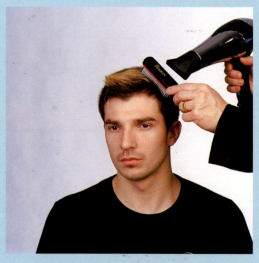

Blow-dry using a Classic Styling Brush and nozzle attachment on dryer.

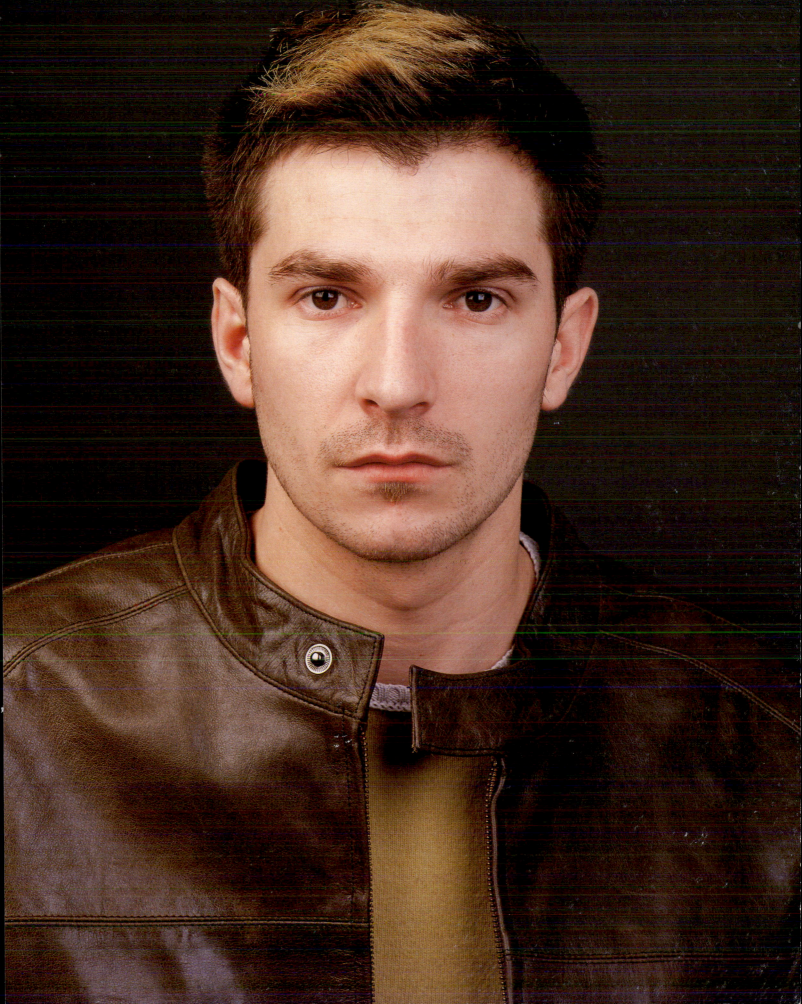

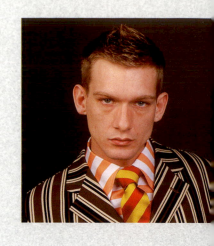

Etonian

COLLECTION

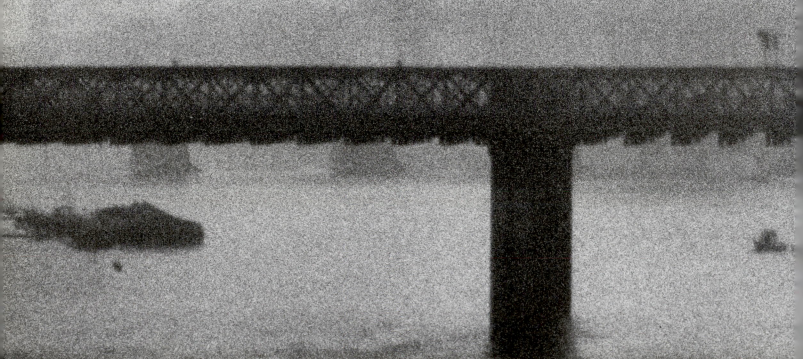

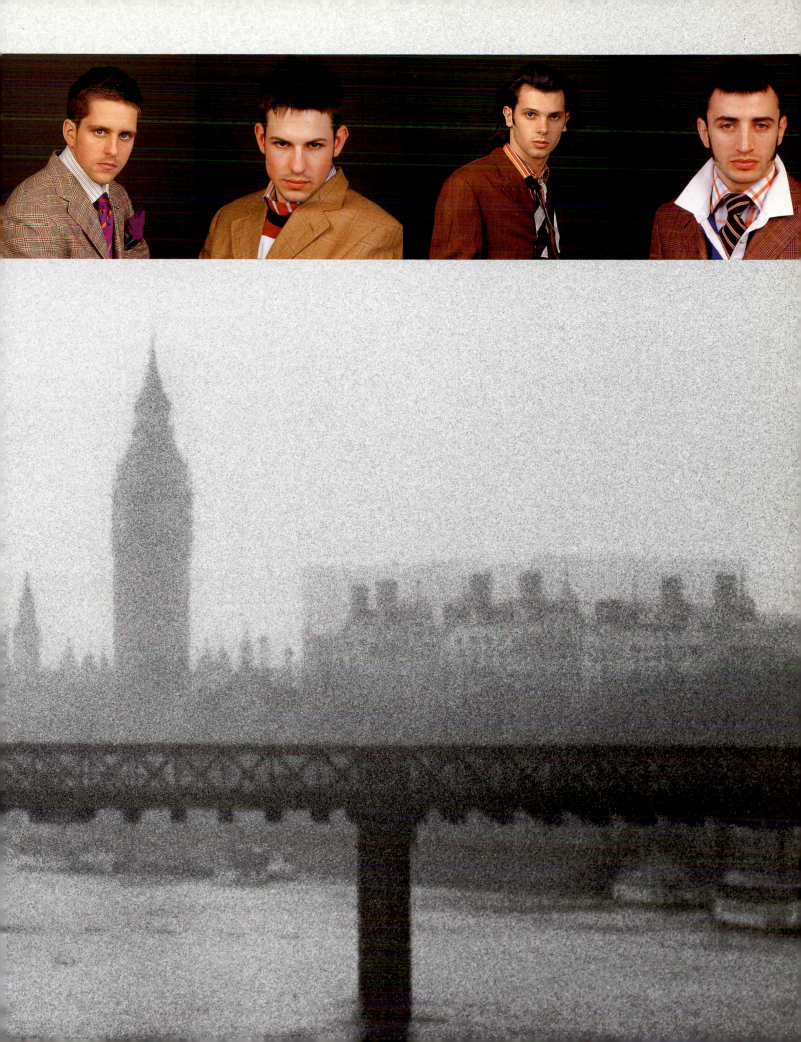

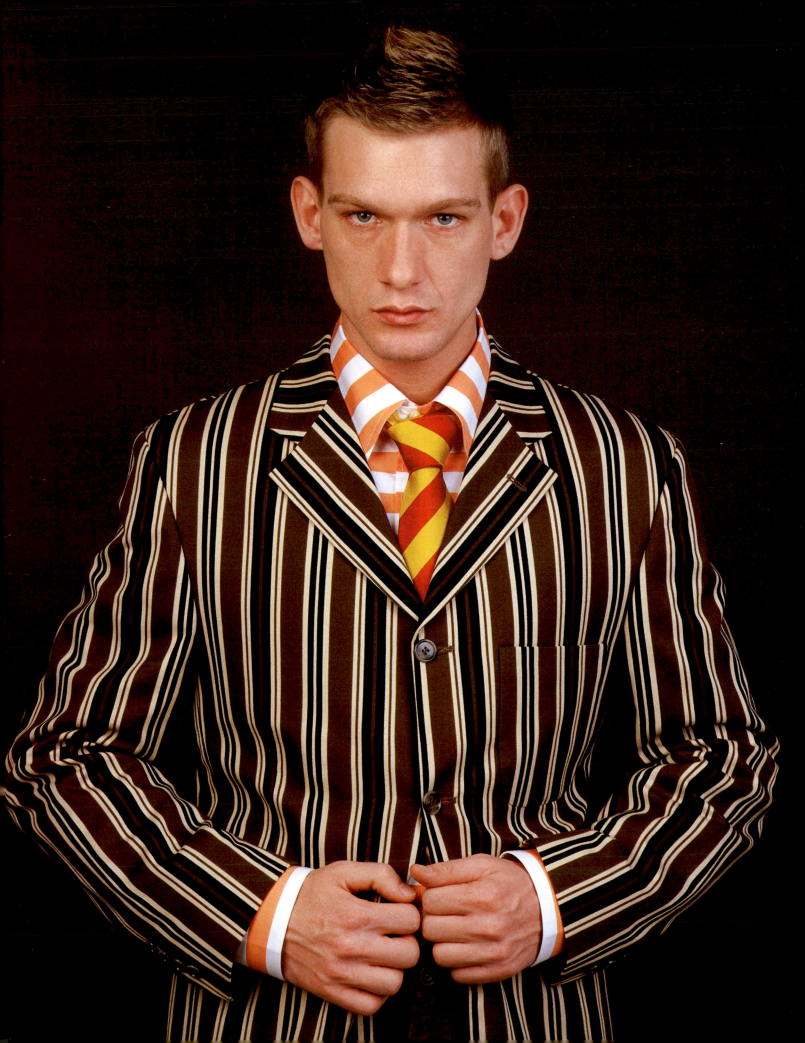

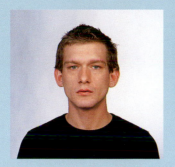

PETER

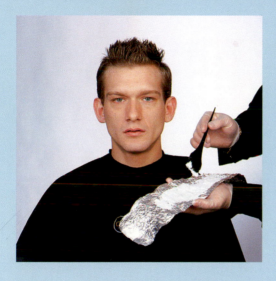

Brush hair upwards. Apply Platine Precision pre-lightening powder (1 scoop + 45ml of 30 vol (9%) L'Oréal Professionnel Cream Oxidant) to a piece of scrunched foil.

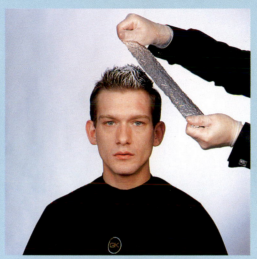

Apply to ends of hair using 'shoe shine' method. Leave to process then rinse thoroughly and shampoo.

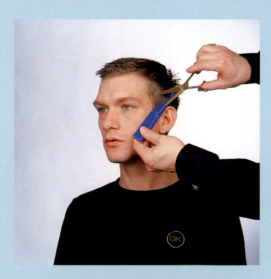

Work on side section using comb and thinning scissors to remove weight and length but retain texture.

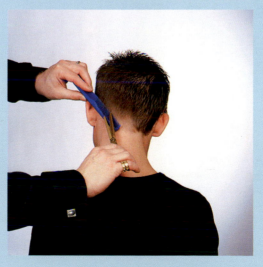

Proceed to back working up from nape area using same method of cutting.

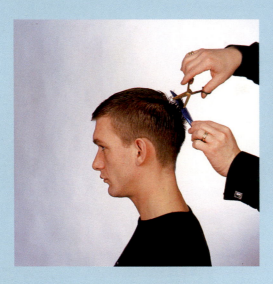

Cut crown hair using a larger comb, elevating hair, removing weight and length.

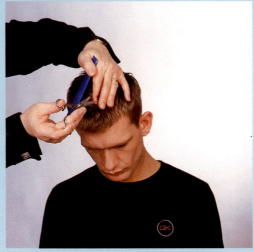

Use scissors to point cut and texturise top.

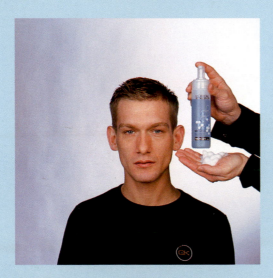

Dispense tecni.art airpump (approximately 4 pumps) into palm of hand.

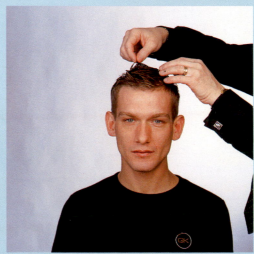

Work product through hair from roots massaging into hair forming the front into a mini quiff. Finish with a little tecni.art Gloss polish.

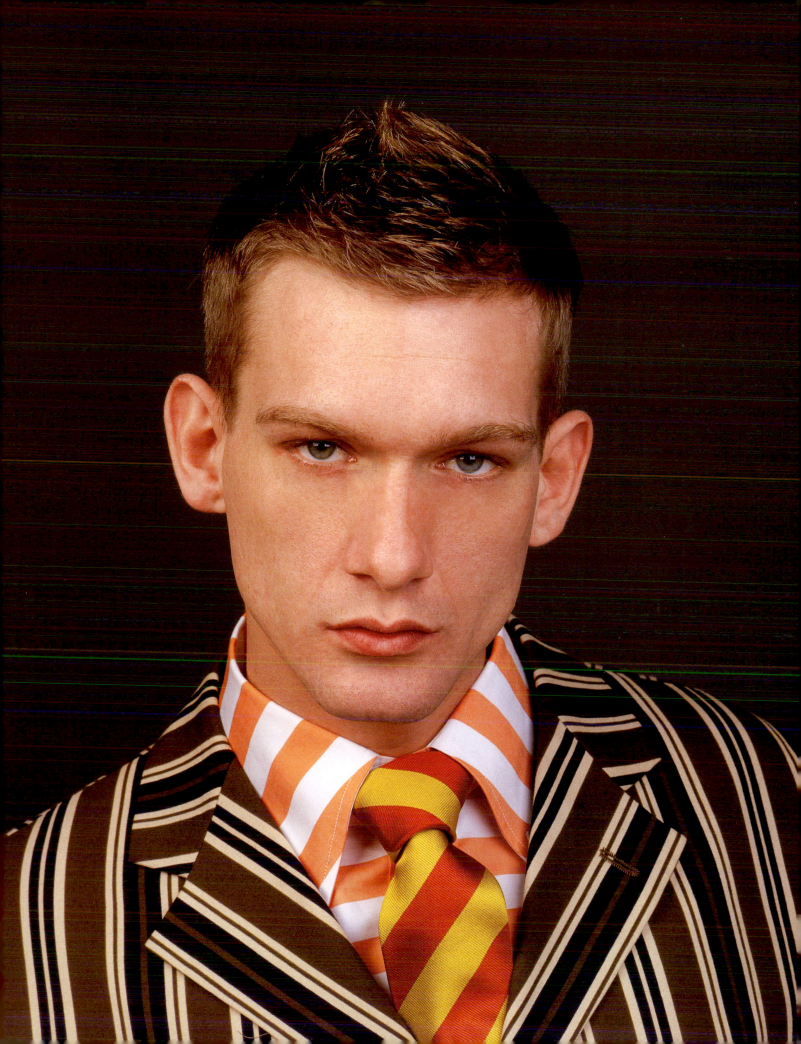

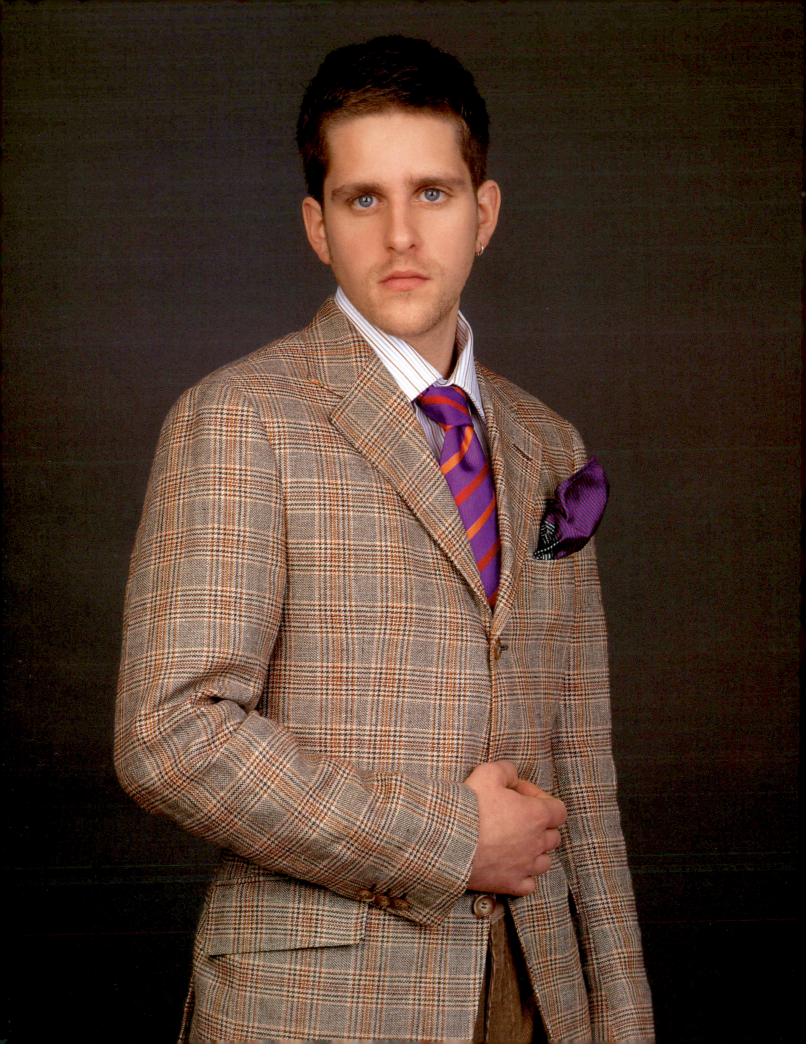

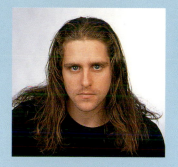

TOM

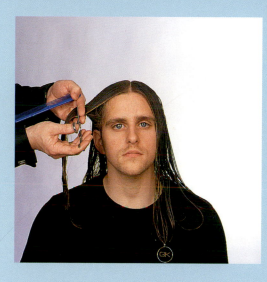

From a centre parting section down to top of ear and remove unwanted length.

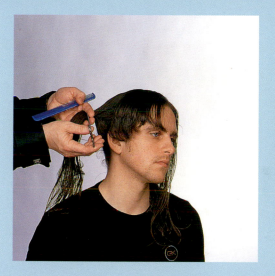

Once guideline is set, cut next section. Then work round back and other side in same manner.

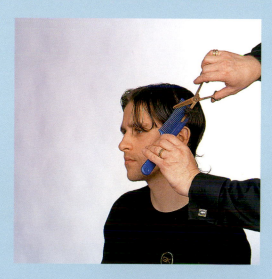

Use thinning scissors over large comb to blend into guideline at side.

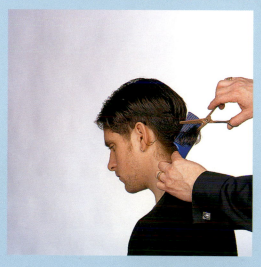

Follow the same method to cut the back and other side section.

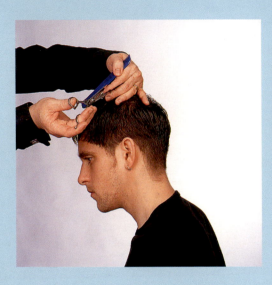

Lift section of crown hair between fingers and use scissors to 'chip into' to shorten length and give a 'fish tail' texture.

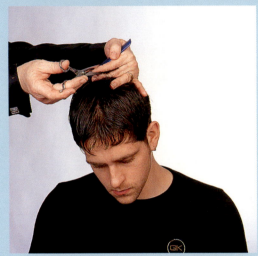

Repeat through crown area.

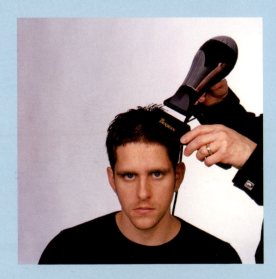

Blow-dry using diffuser attachment and a Paddle Brush.

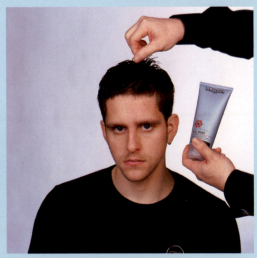

Sculpt and fix hair achieving that 'messed-up' look using tecni.art Fix max, working into hair with fingers, where required.

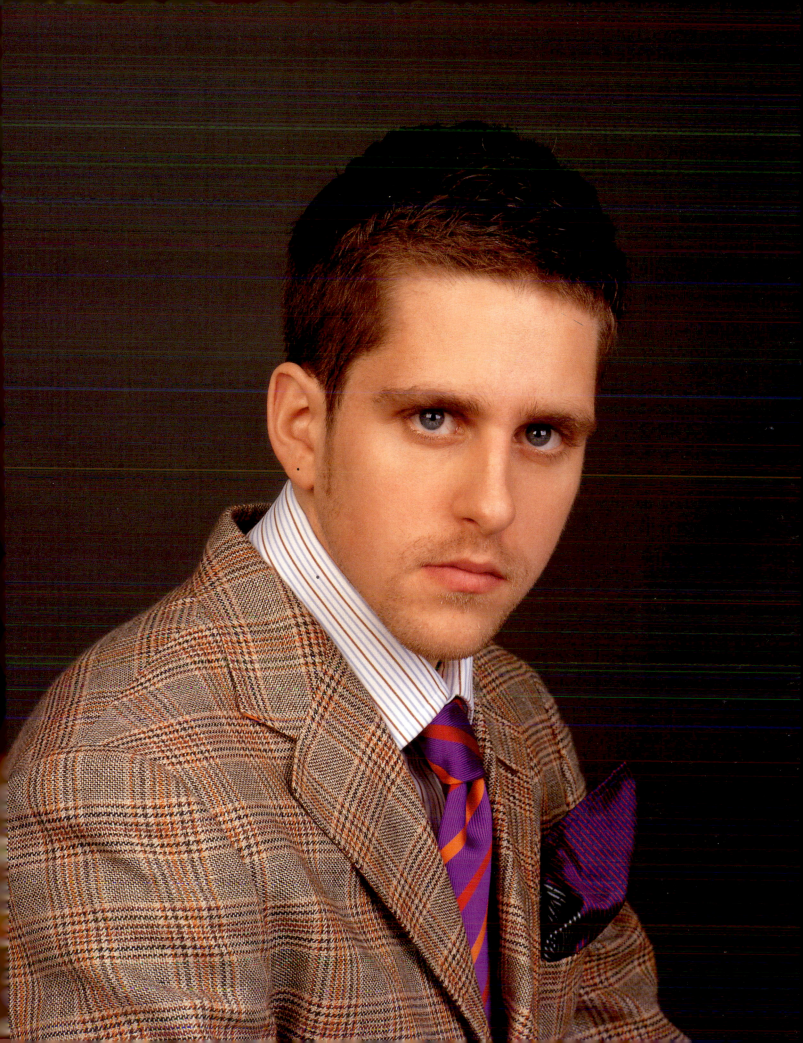

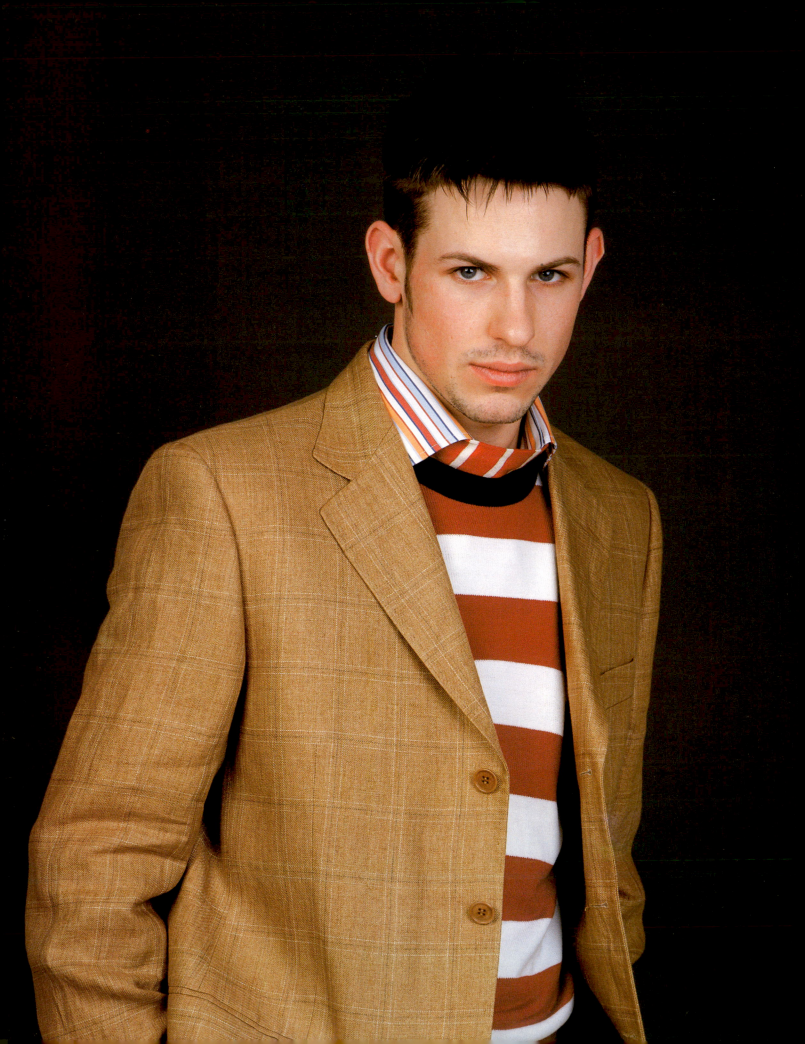

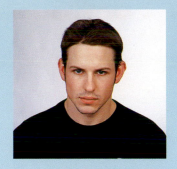

BARRY

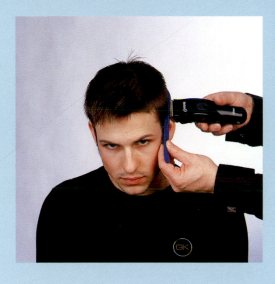

Work on side sections using clipper over comb to achieve close cut.

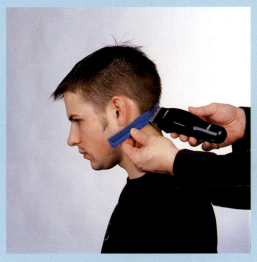

Continue in same manner at back working from nape up to crown.

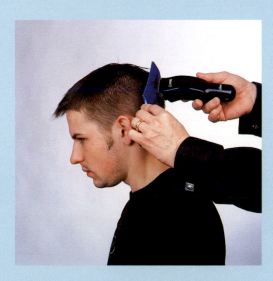

Using a larger comb, clipper cut from base of comb upwards.

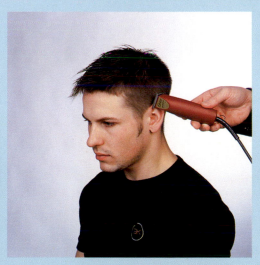

Use finisher clipper to clean round ear.

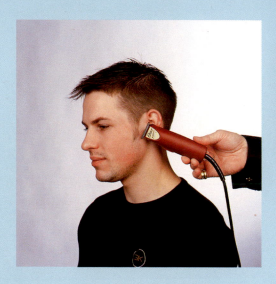

Neaten and clean up sideburn.

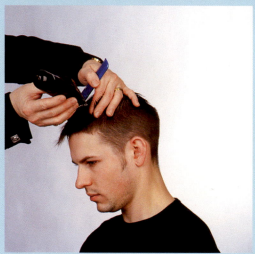

Use clippers to chip into crown hair.

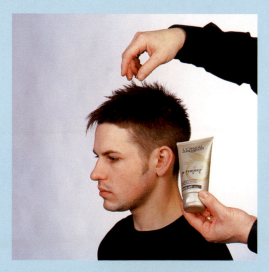

Work tecni.art a-head GLUE into ends of hair to sculpt and give that messed-up look.

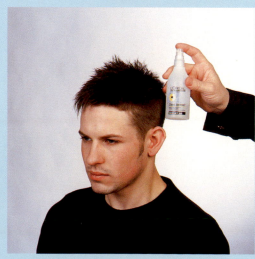

Mist with tecni.art Gloss control to give hold and shine.

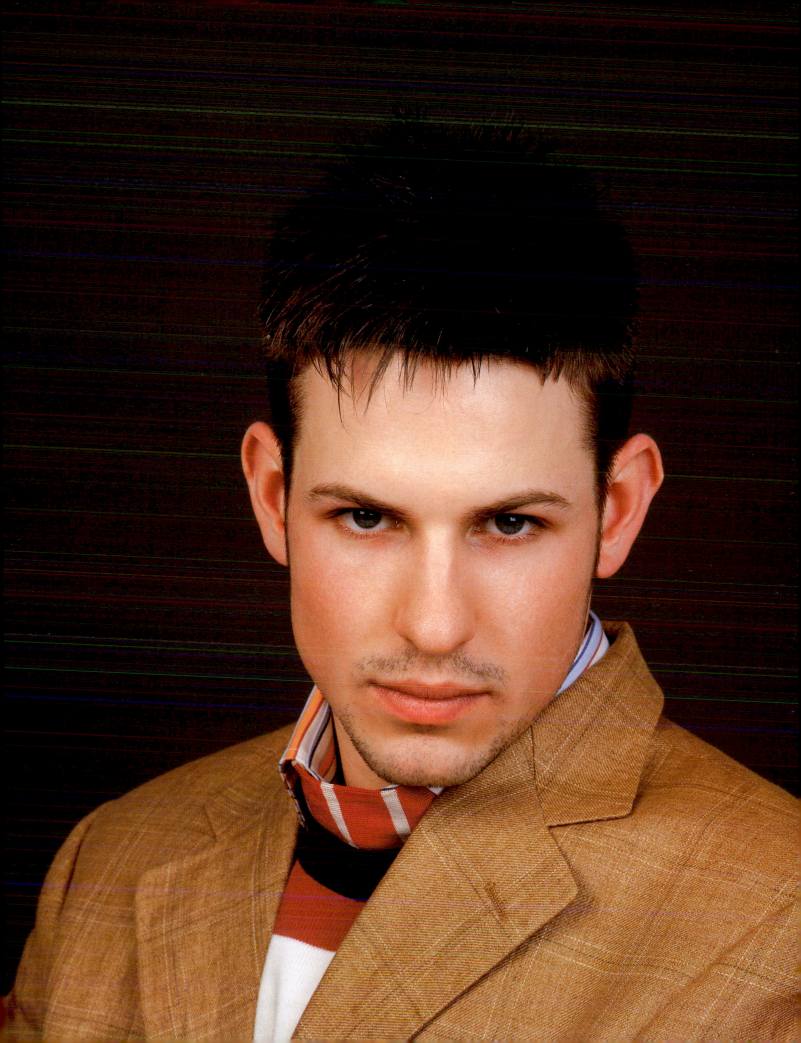

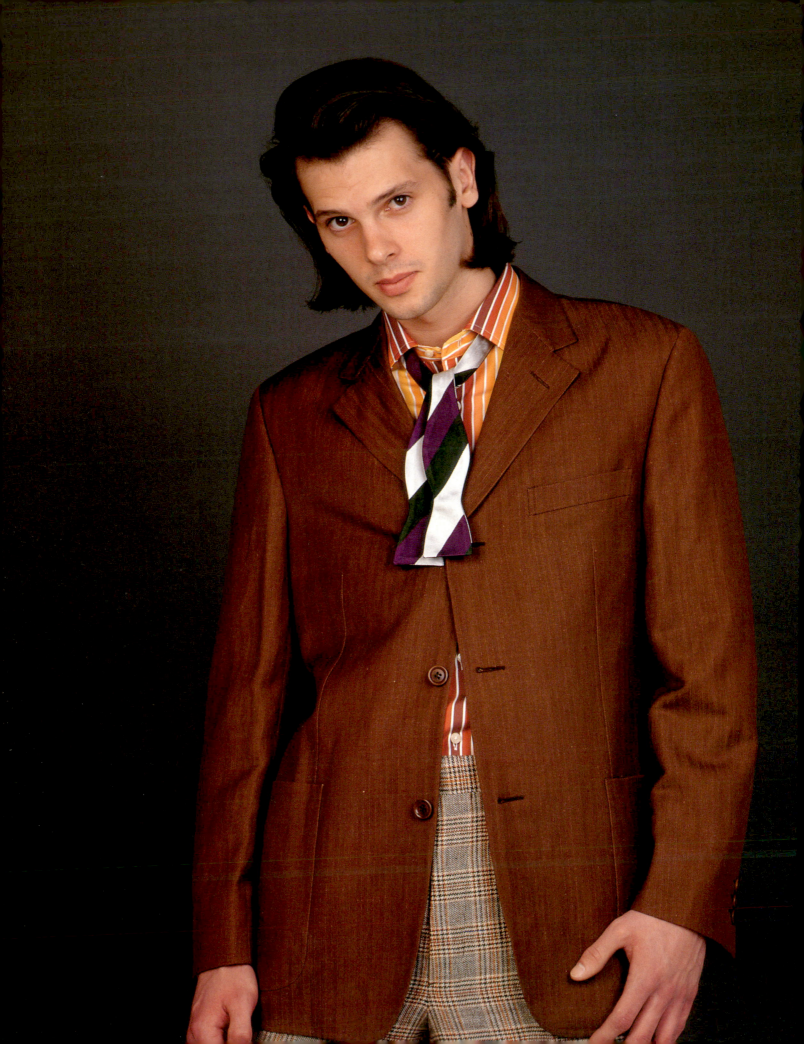

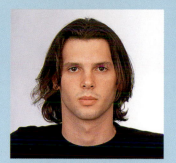

SHAUN

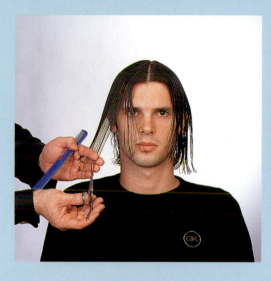

From a centre parting take side section and point cut end 1.5cm.

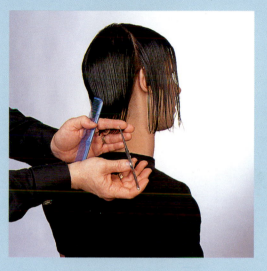

Point cut back and side section in same way and then other side.

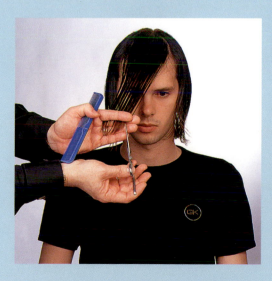

Take a triangular section at front and overdirect hair forward. Point cut ends removing 1.5cm of length.

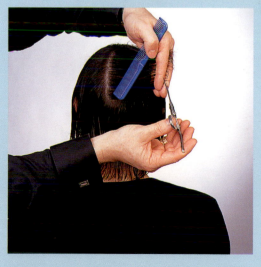

Take a vertical section from centre of head to occipital bone. Point cut into ends removing 1cm of length. Work forward from each side in same manner.

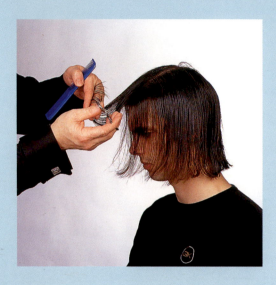

Take central section and blend holding hair firmly in hand whilst working.

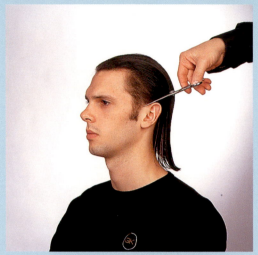

Trim round sideburns and clean up round ears.

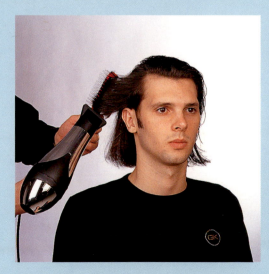

Apply tecni.art Volume + to give control and softness then use a Classic Styling Brush to dry hair section by section.

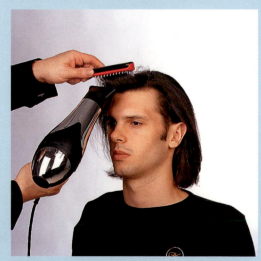

Create quiff by pushing roots forward at front thus achieving just the right amount of lift. Mist with tecni.art Airfix to hold the style.

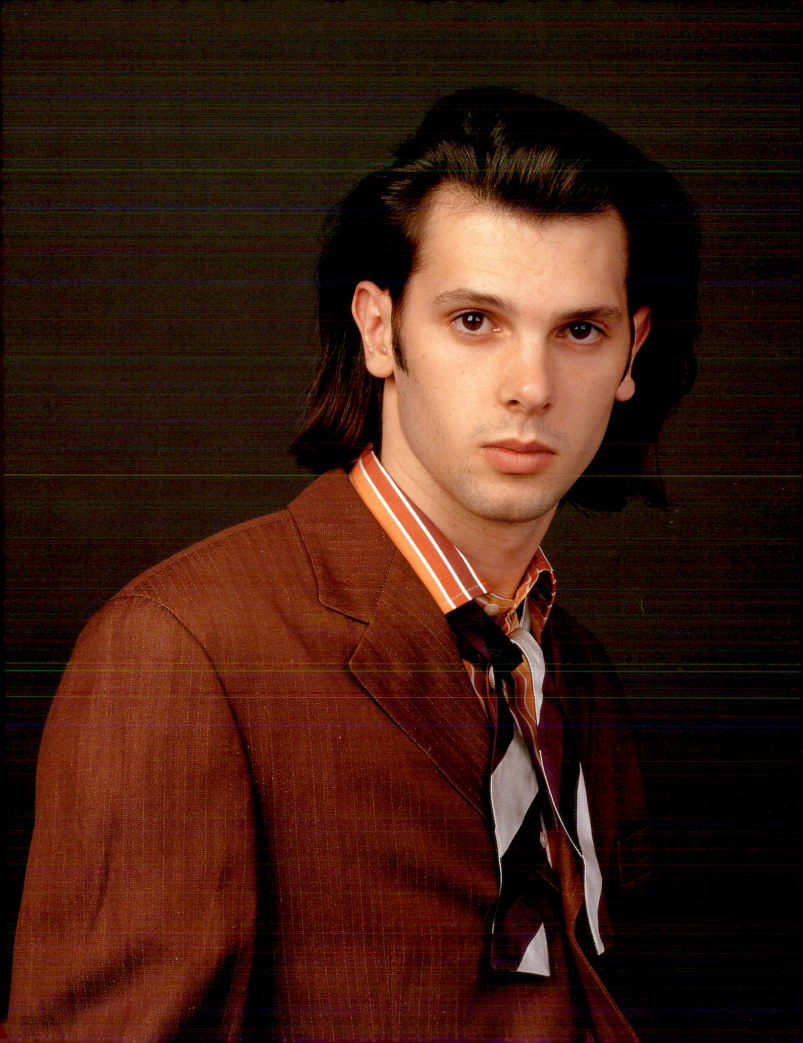

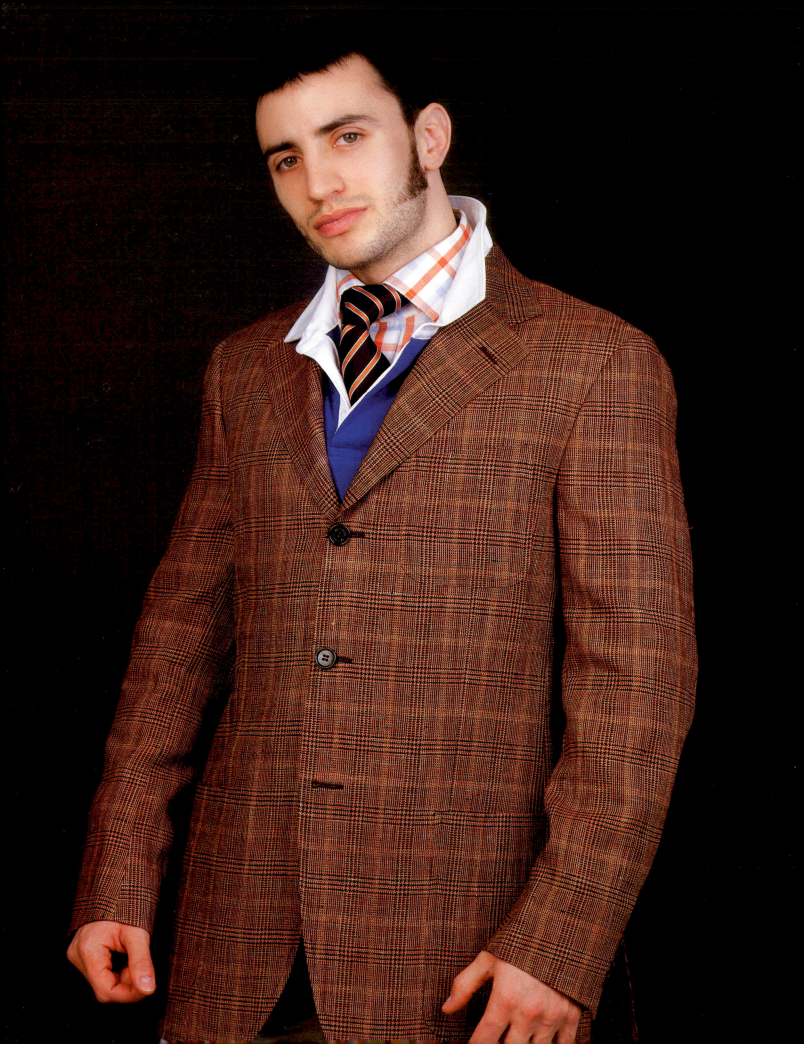

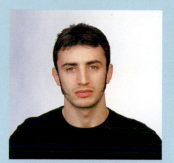

SILVIU

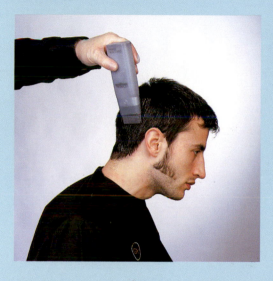

To cover the first signs of grey we used L'Oréal Professionnel Diacolor homme. Mix following instructions, and apply colour using the STAC applicator bottle working from nape upwards.

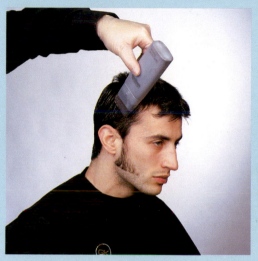

Continue in this manner, up towards crown, applying several times.

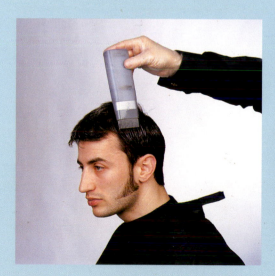

Work on other side in same way.

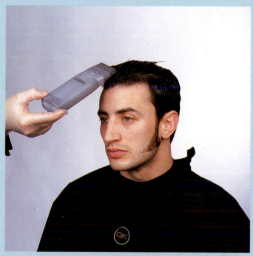

Finally apply colour to crown area. Leave to develop for 15 minutes then emulsify, rinse thoroughly and shampoo.

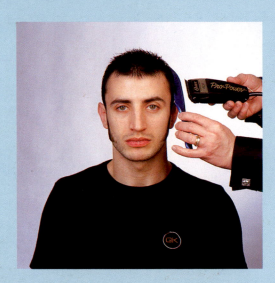

Cut sides using clipper over comb to remove length.

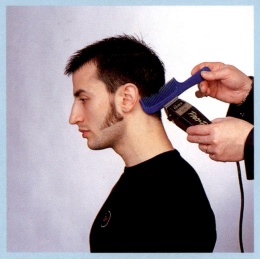

Work from nape up towards occipital bone in same manner, combing upwards and cutting from base of comb. Hold comb at same angle throughout.

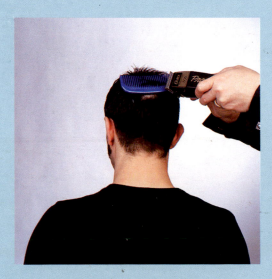

Remove length from crown using clipper over comb.

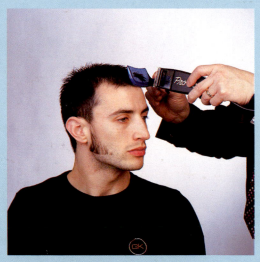

Point cut fringe using clipper over comb. Finish hair using tecni.art Aqua gloss to give a wet look tousled finish.

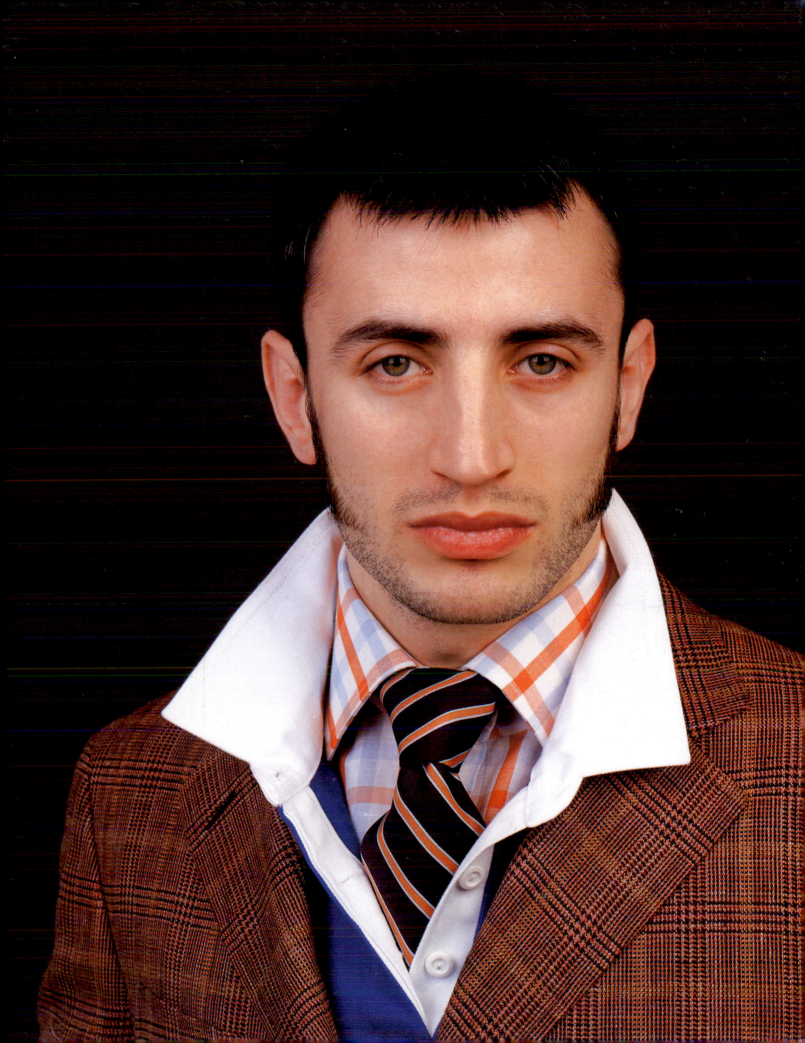

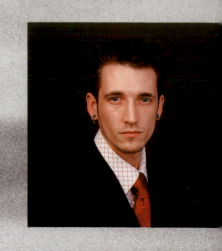

City

COLLECTION

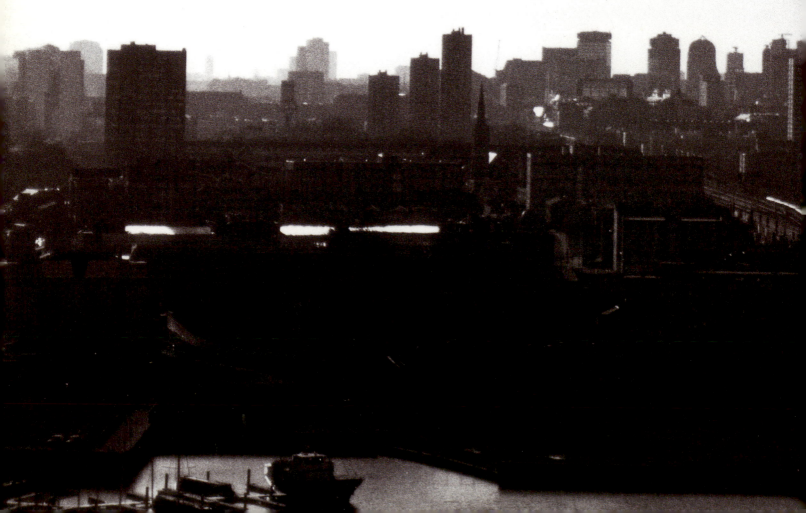

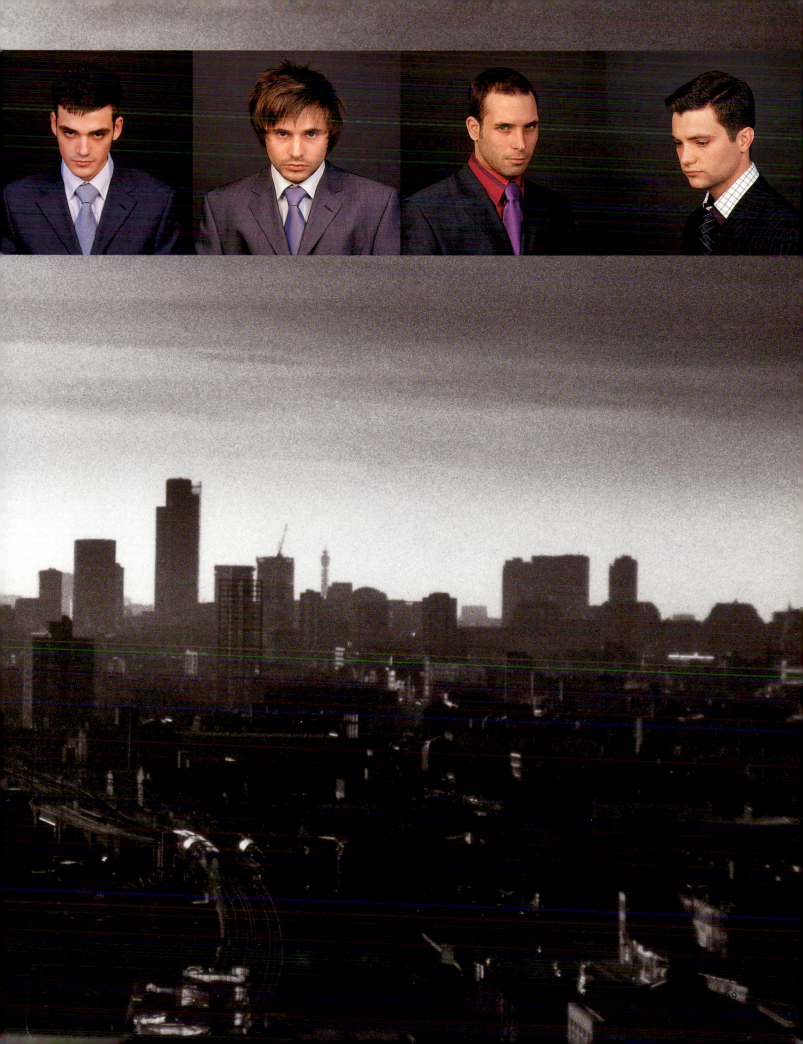

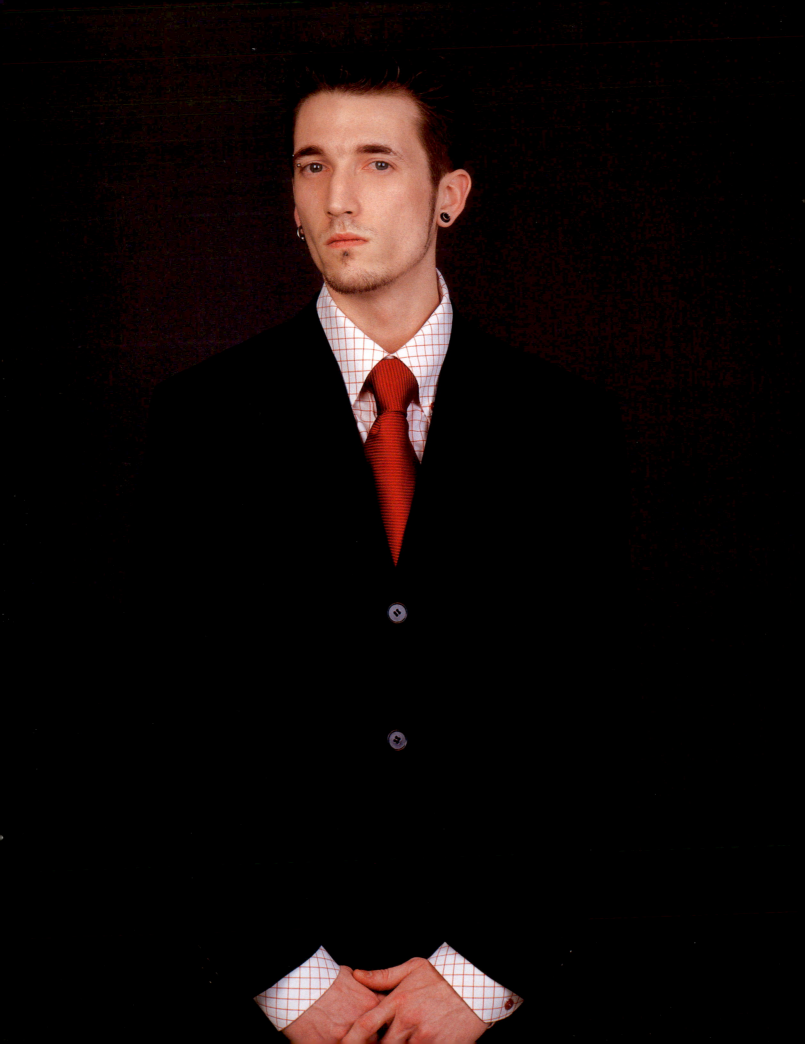

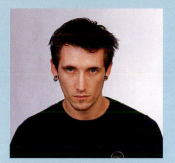

GUILLAUME

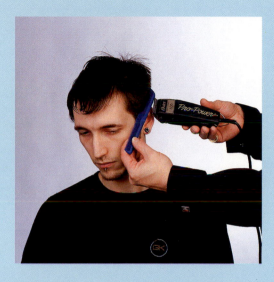

Using freehand elevation work clipper over fine end of comb on side.

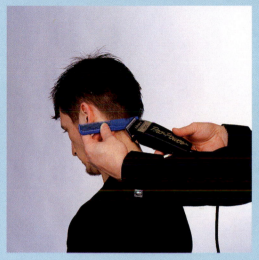

Work from nape to occipital bone in the same manner.

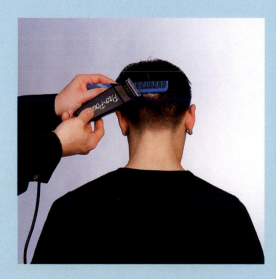

Switch to wide end of comb and clipper back area.

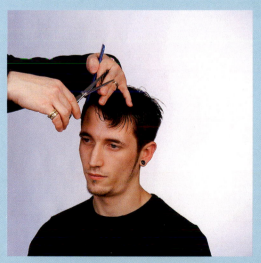

Take vertical sections of front hair and cut 1.5cm to reduce length.

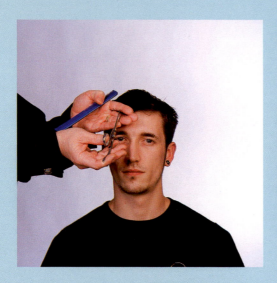

Point cut front area.

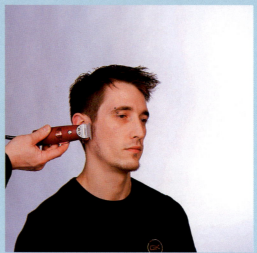

Use a finisher clipper to clean up round sideburns.

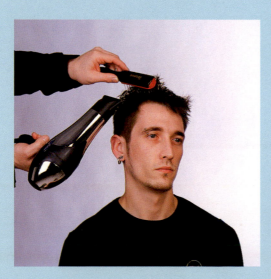

With nozzle attachment on the dryer use a Classic Brush to dry hair lifting away from roots as you dry.

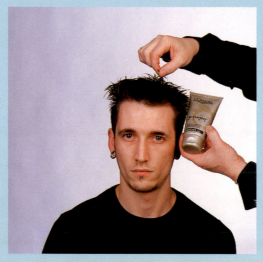

Apply tecni.art a-head GLUE to ends of hair to give subtle texture.

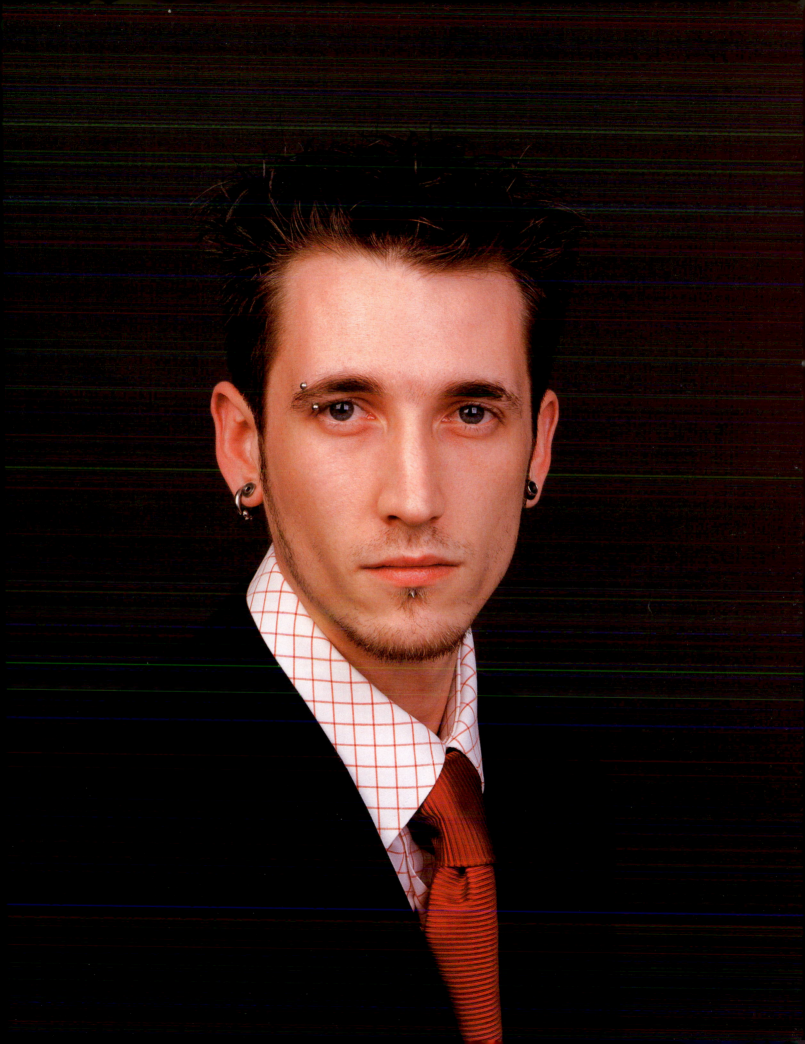

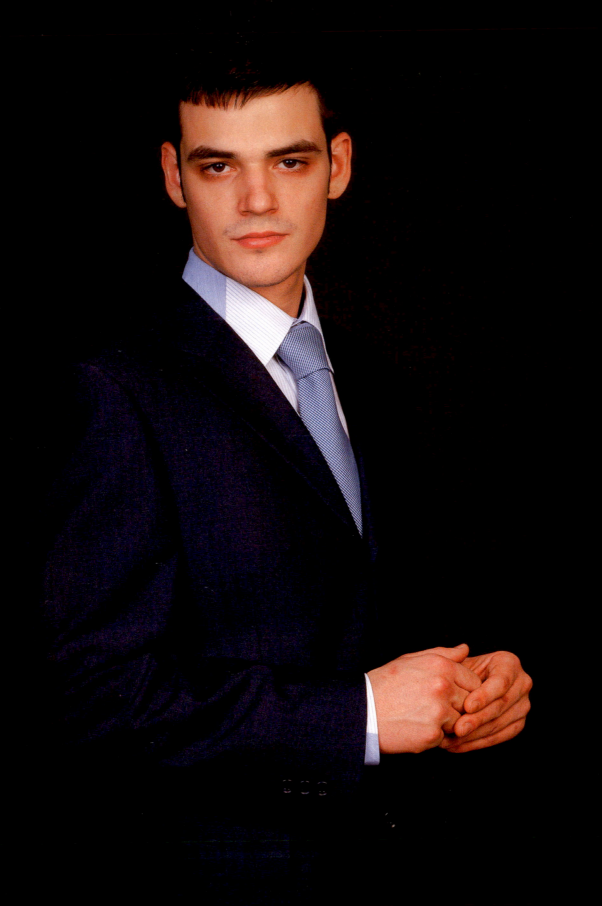

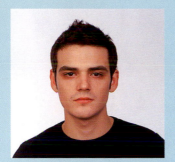

PHILIP

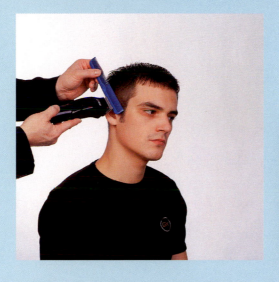

Using fine side of comb, work freehand, clipper over comb, cutting to desired length.

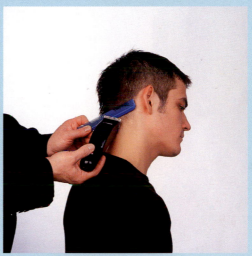

Cut nape hair in same way.

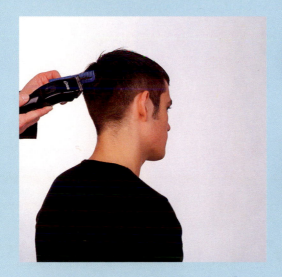

Switch to wider end of comb, continue with freehand clipper technique and work up back of head to occipital bone.

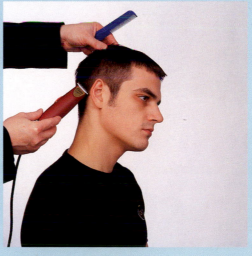

Use finisher clipper to clean up round sideburns and ears.

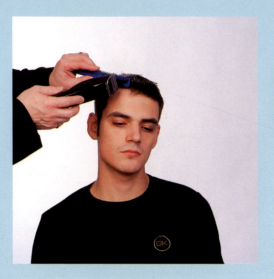

Point cut into hairline using clipper over wider end of comb.

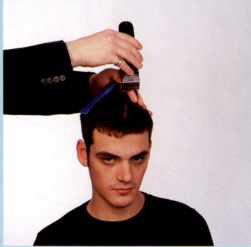

Take vertical sections on crown and 'chip into' using clipper.

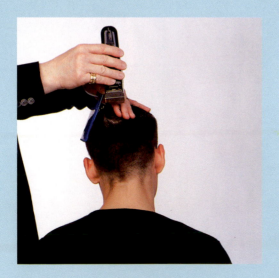

Blend crown hair by point cutting with clipper.

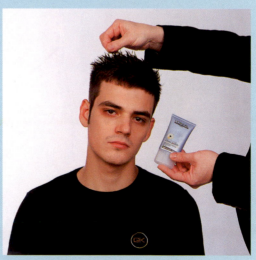

Add a shiny polished effect using tecni.art Gloss polish applied with fingers.

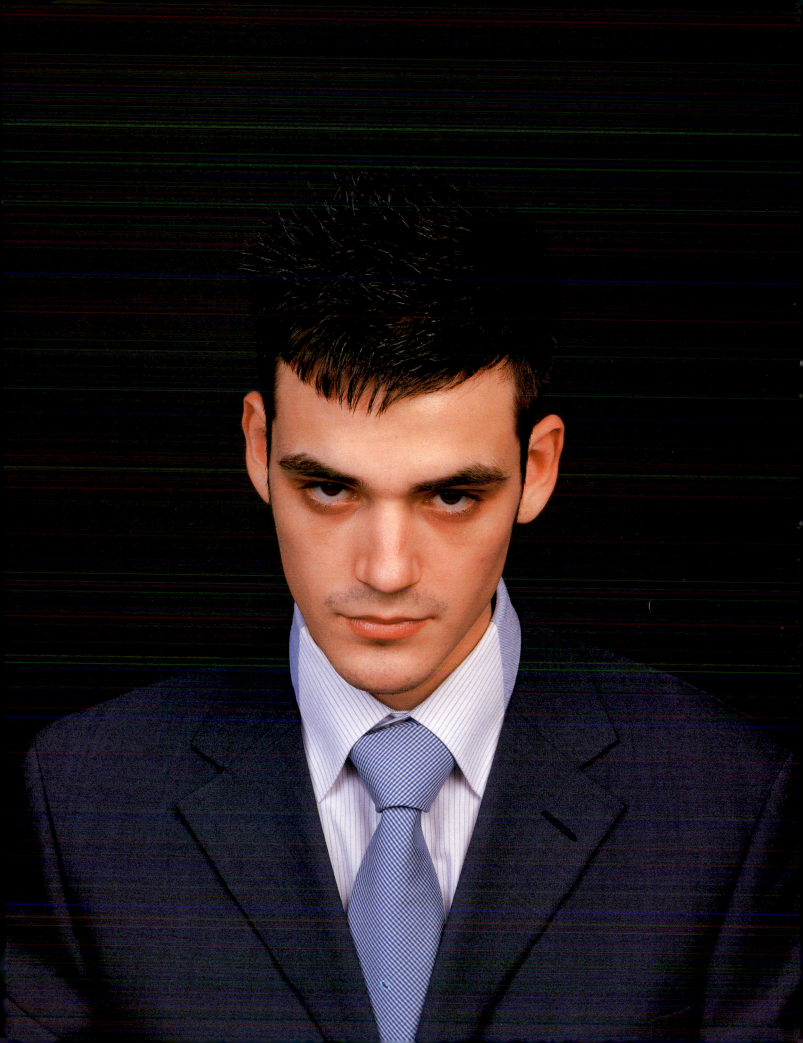

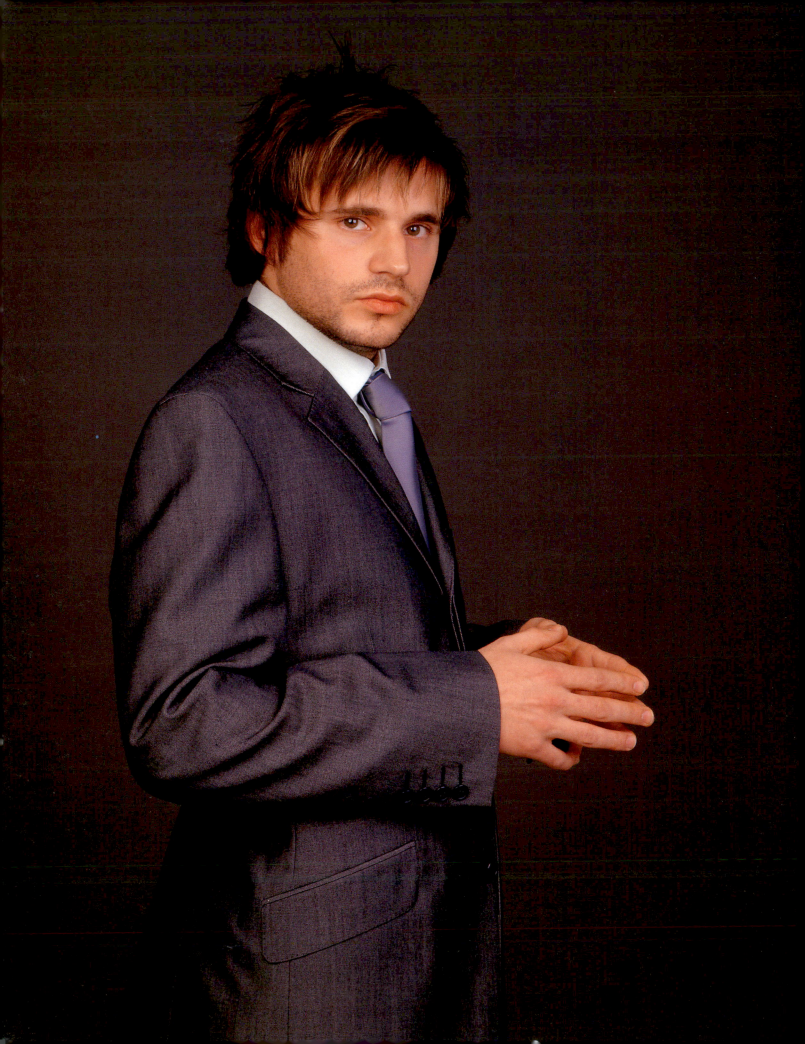

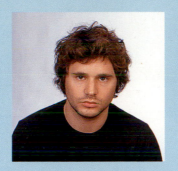

JAMES

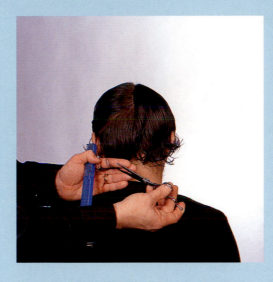

Part down centre back then diagonally to ear.
Remove 2cm of length. Repeat on other side.

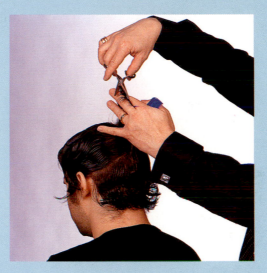

Remove 2cm from top section working from
centre parting towards ear thus reducing weight.

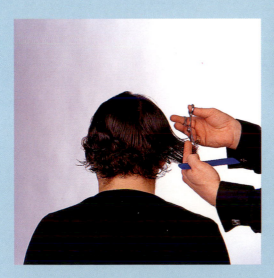

For the last section, before cutting, overdirect the
hair.

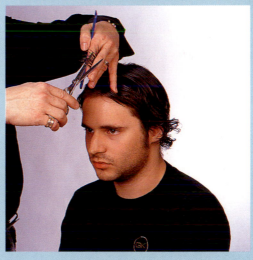

From a centre parting take a vertical elevation and
remove 2cm of length.

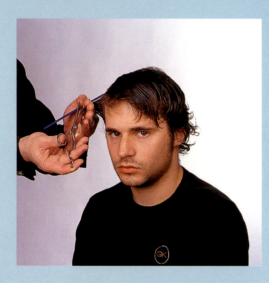

Take a vertical section from side to top of ear, slightly over directing forward. Point cut to remove length and create texture.

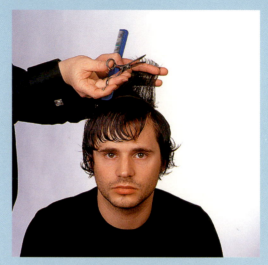

From a side parting take top section and point cut to texturise.

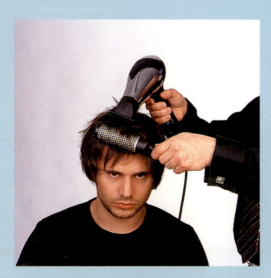

Use Hot Curl Brush to give smoothness whilst drying with nozzle attachment on dryer.

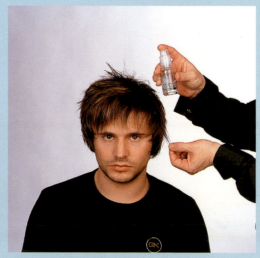

Work tecni.art Liss Control + into hair to help prevent it from going frizzy and to maintain blow-dry finish smooth.

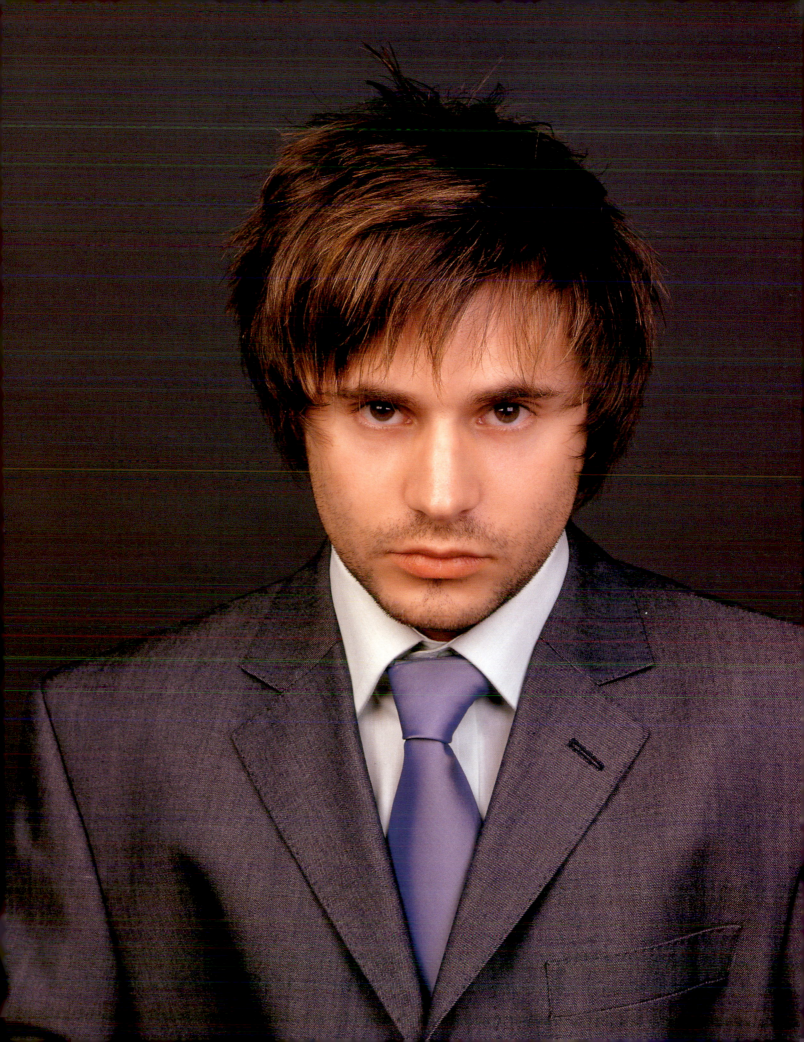

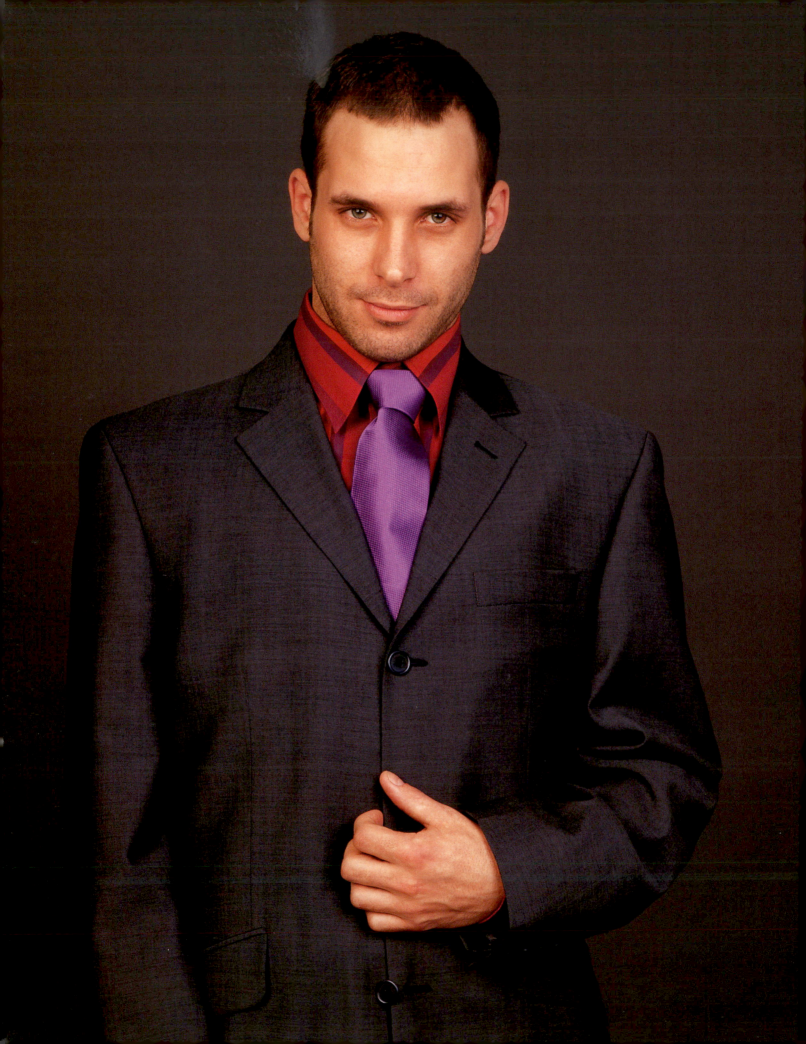

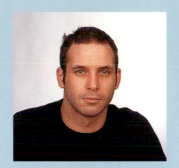

DAMIEN

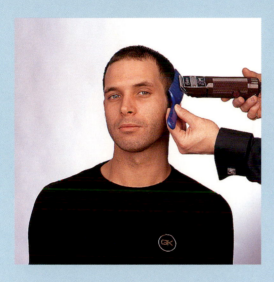

Work clipper over comb from ear to temple.

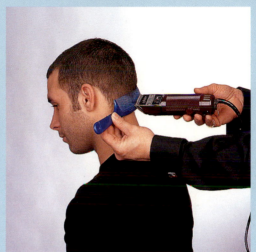

Proceed in the same way from nape area up to occipital bone.

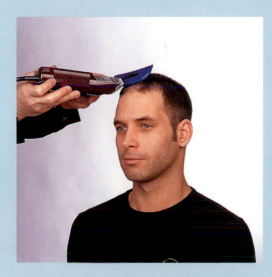

Work from hairline to crown, clipper over comb.

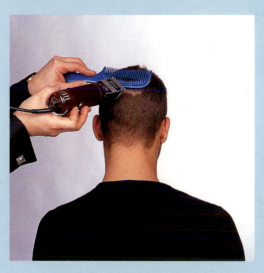

Then proceed to back and crown area

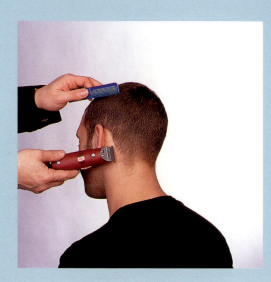

Clean up nape using finisher clipper.

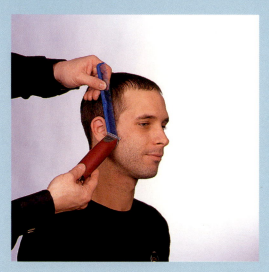

Neaten sideburns using finisher clipper.

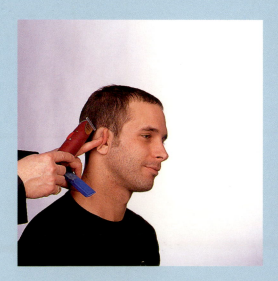

Tidy round the ears.

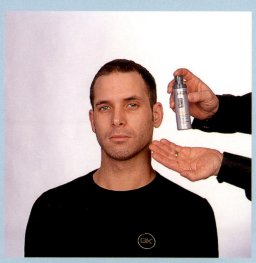

Dispense tecni.art Gloss boost onto the palm of the hands and work through hair for maximum shine.

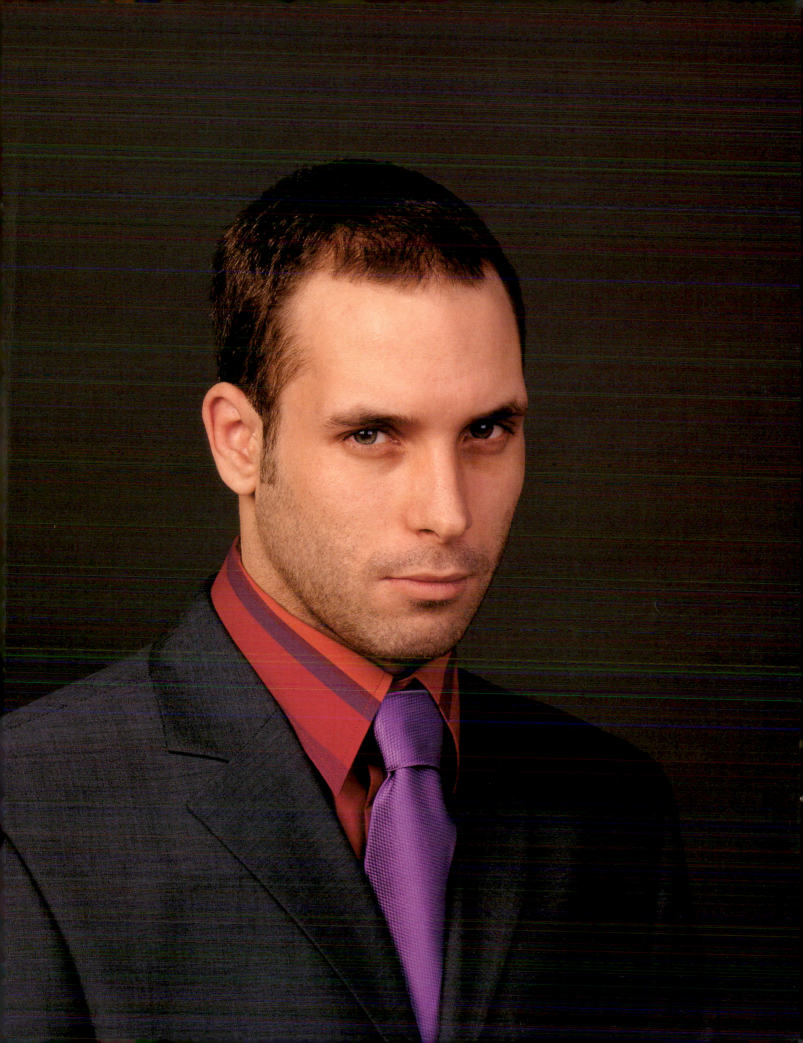

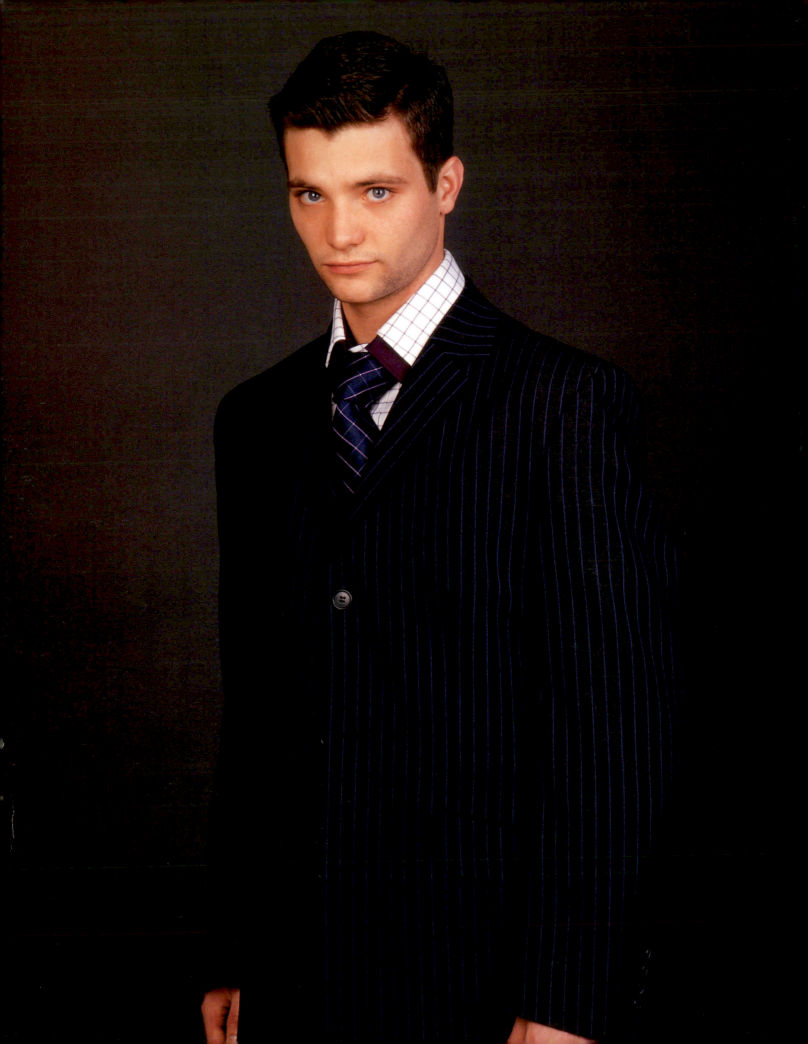

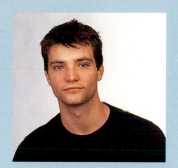

HECTOR

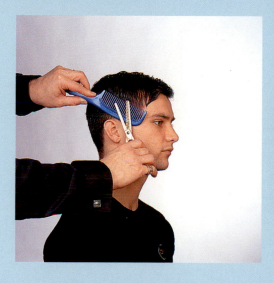

Use thinning scissors over comb working from ear to temple.

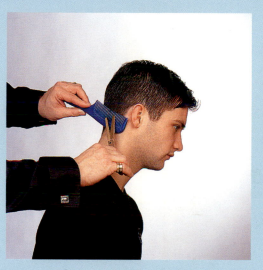

Work from the nape of neck upwards in same manner.

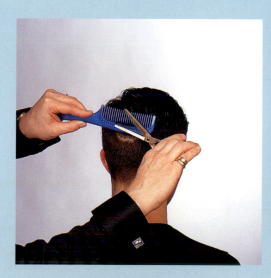

Cut back hair using freehand elevation and thinning scissors over comb.

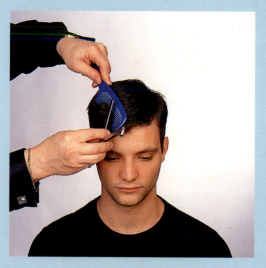

Use razor over comb to remove weight and length.

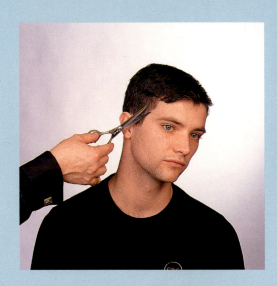

Clean up round sides and hairline using scissors.

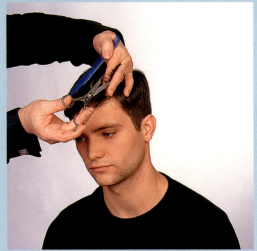

Point cut top section with scissors to create texture.

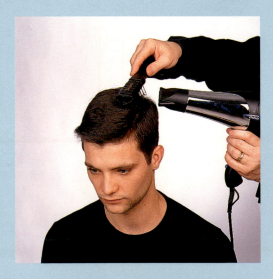

Dry using a Tunnel Vent Brush to get root lift.

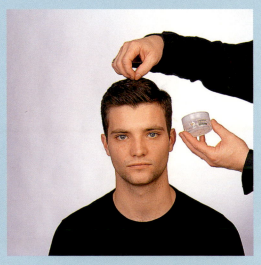

Apply tecni.art Digit gloss section by section to finish.

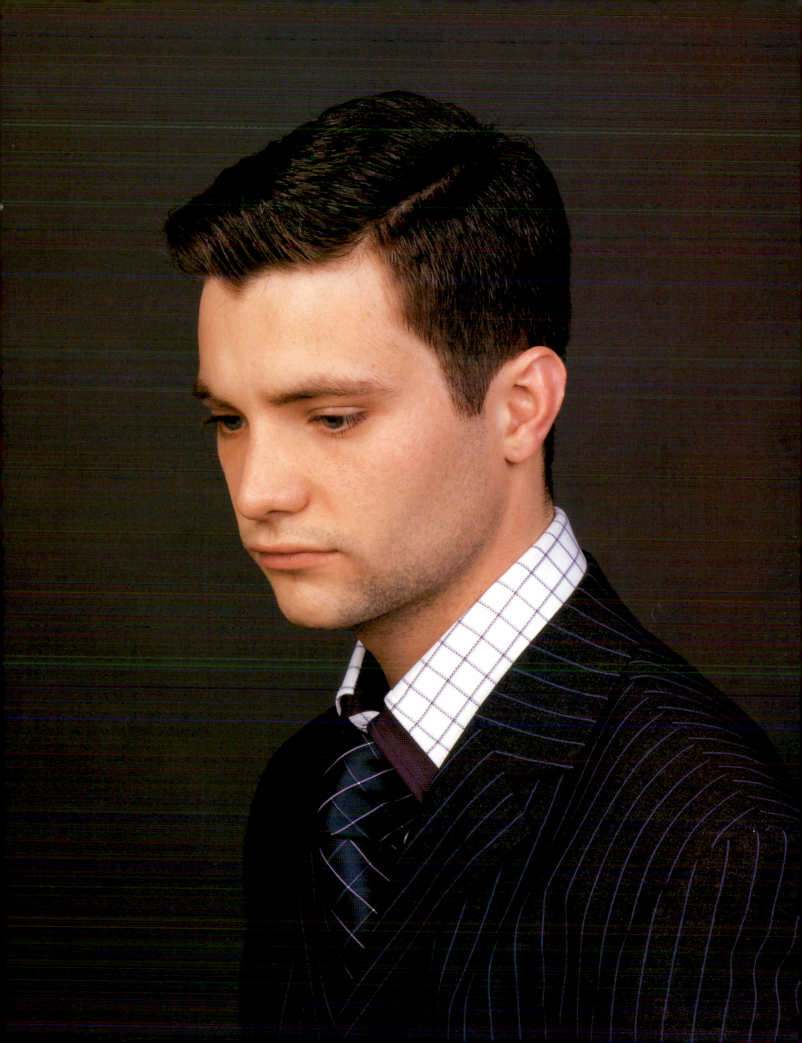

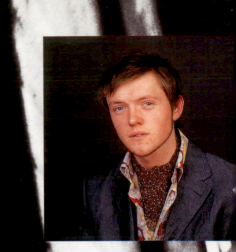

Bohemian

COLLECTION

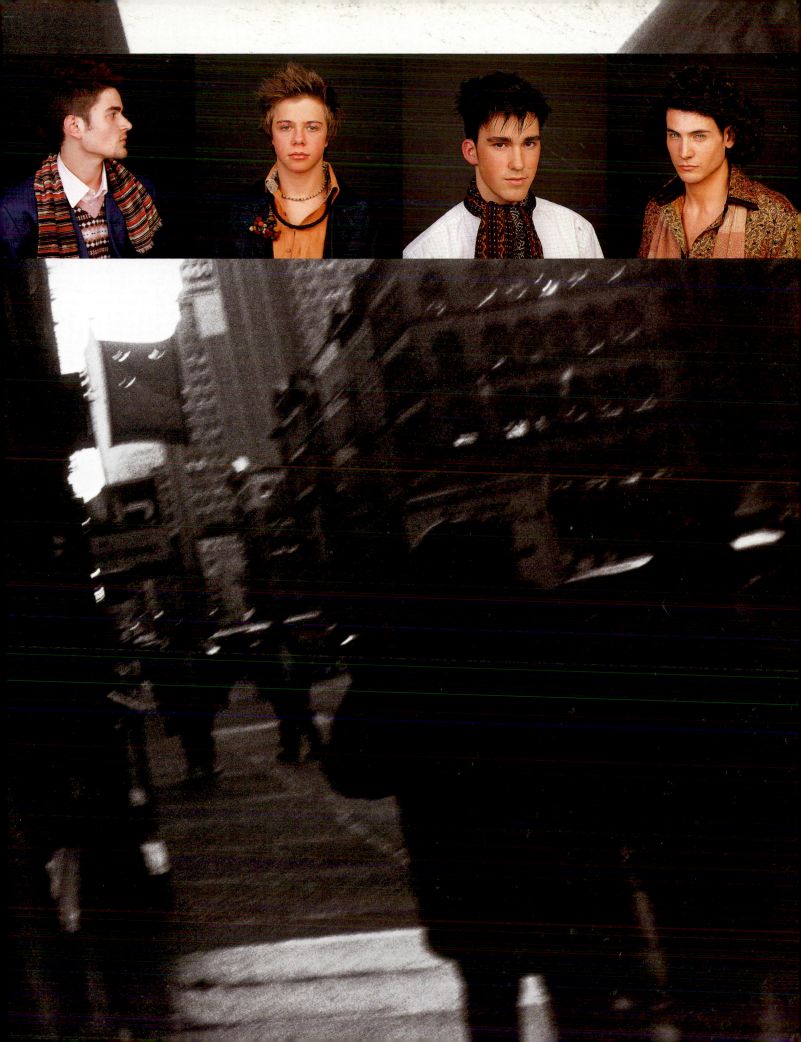

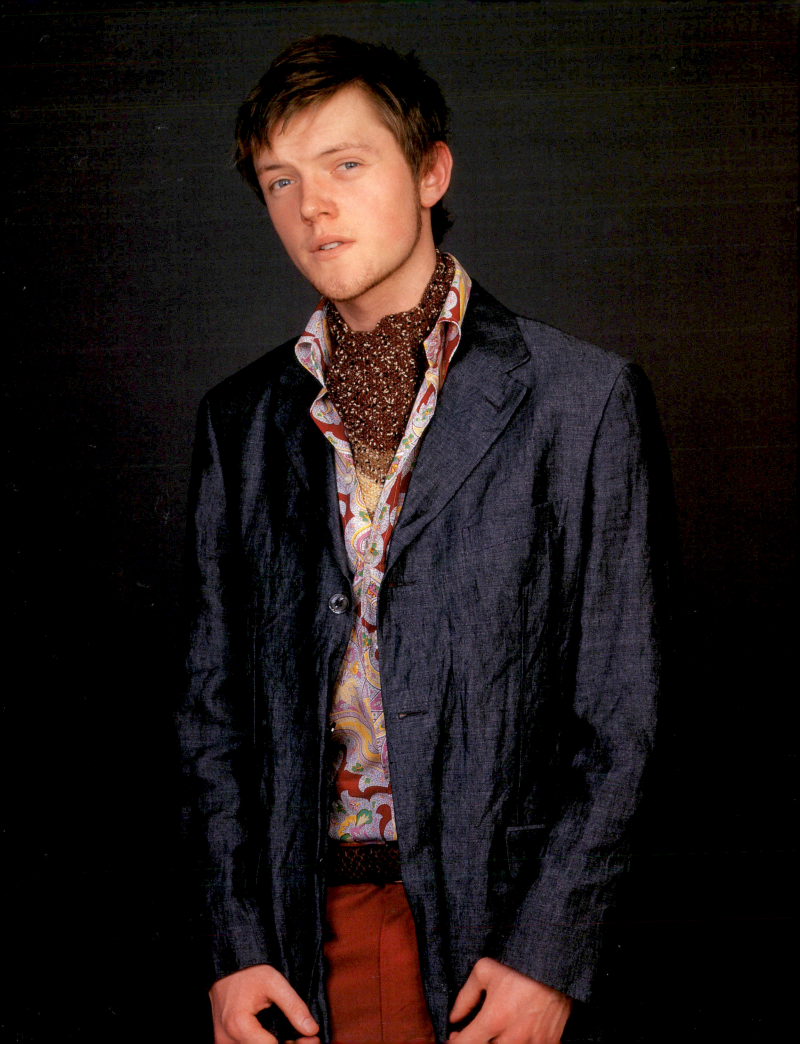

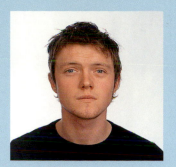

TOM

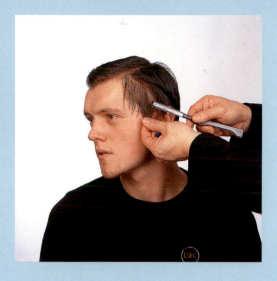

Part hair at side. Take a vertical section from temple to ear and point cut using a razor.

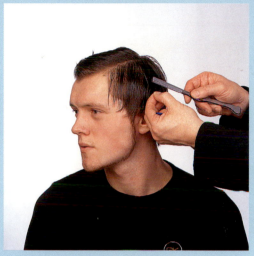

Take next section in the same manner and continue to point cut through side section.

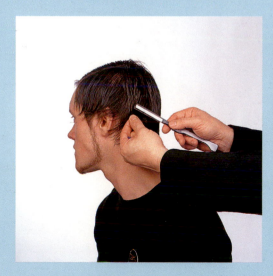

At the back, take a vertical section and overdirect hair, continue using razor technique to remove length and to texturise. Repeat for other side.

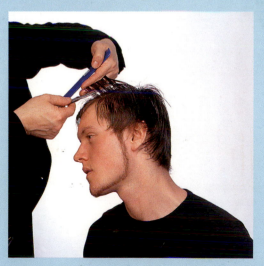

Take section on crown and weave razor in and out 1cm away from roots, move razor towards ends to remove length and weight.

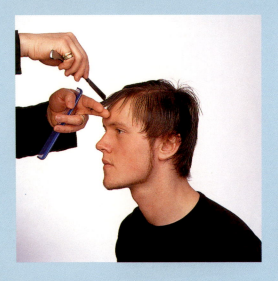

Point cut fringe using razor.

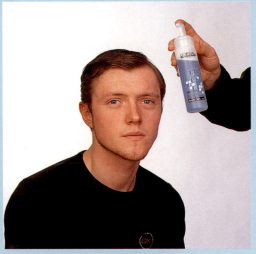

Boost hair and give lift using tecni.art airpump.

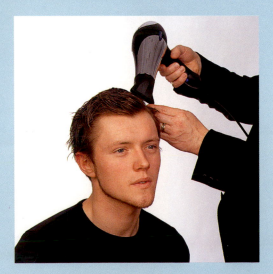

Blow-dry with nozzle attachment lifting hair with fingers.

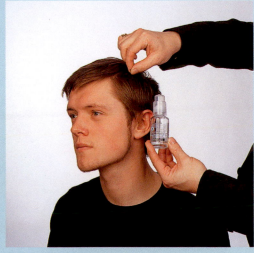

Finish using tecni.art Liss control which defines and protects hair against humidity.

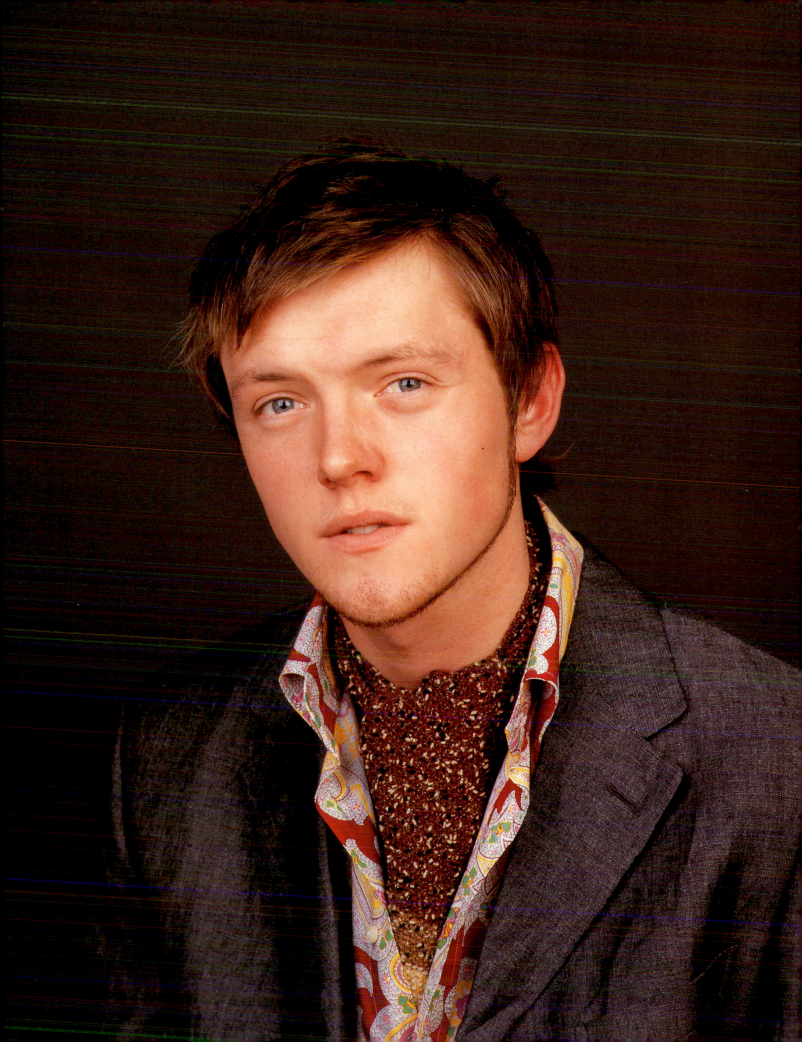

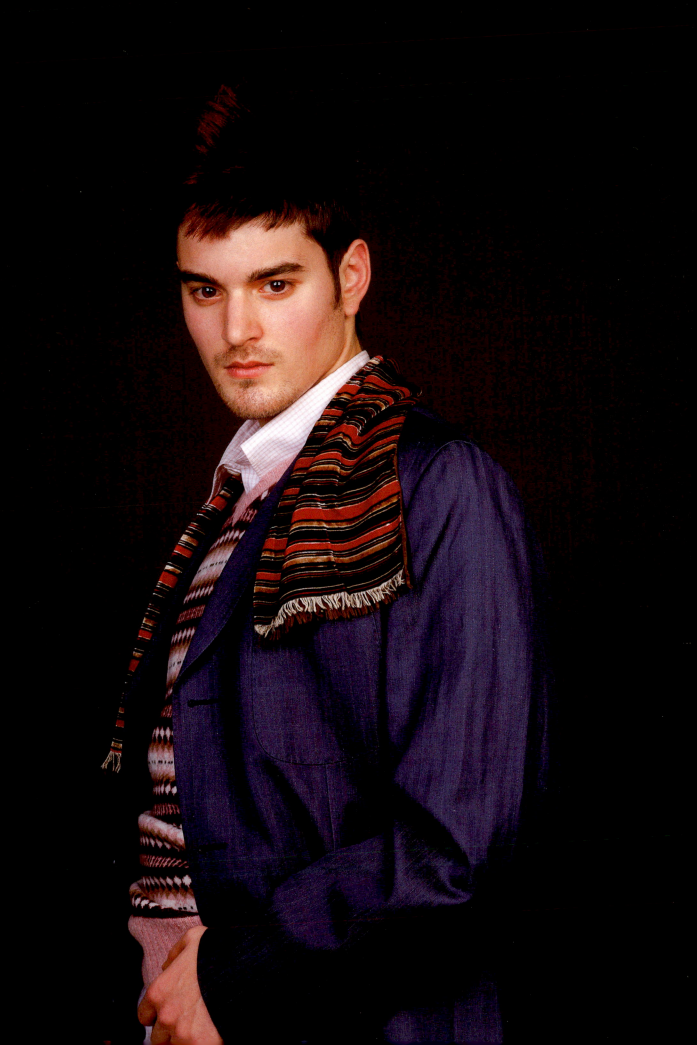

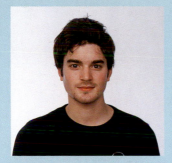

MICHAEL

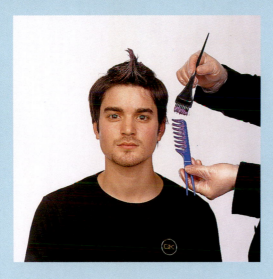

Using Majirouge 6.66 Dark Extra Red Blonde (25ml + 37.5ml 20 vol (6%) L'Oréal Professionnel cream oxidant), apply colour to quiff using wide tooth comb.

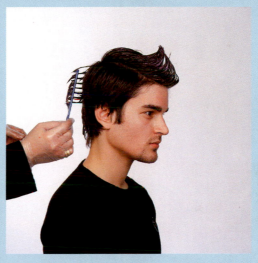

In same manner apply colour to ducks tail at back of head. Leave to develop. To remove, emulsify and shampoo.

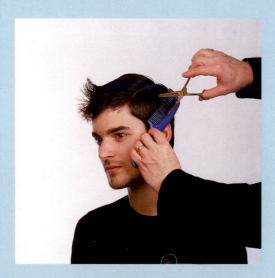

Use wide tooth comb and thinning scissors to remove length and weight at side.

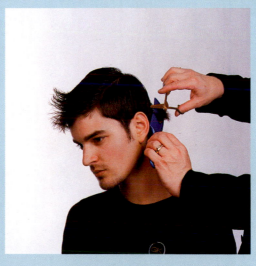

Work upwards from nape in the same manner.

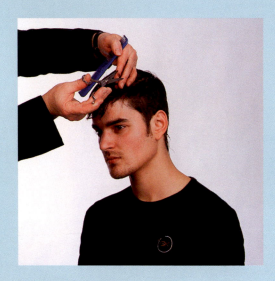

Take a vertical section at crown and point cut to remove length. Proceed through the top area in same manner.

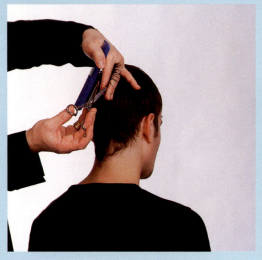

Work on centre back leaving ducks tail section longer but point cutting into it for texture.

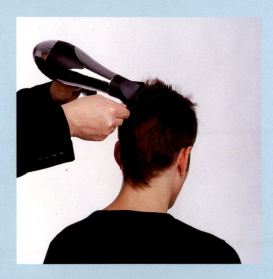

Blow-dry hair using a Paddle Brush.

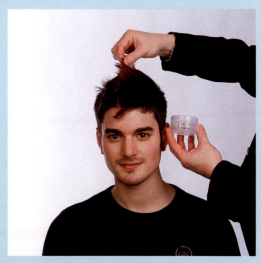

Finish using tecni.art Digit gloss to give maximum shine and a ruffled finish.

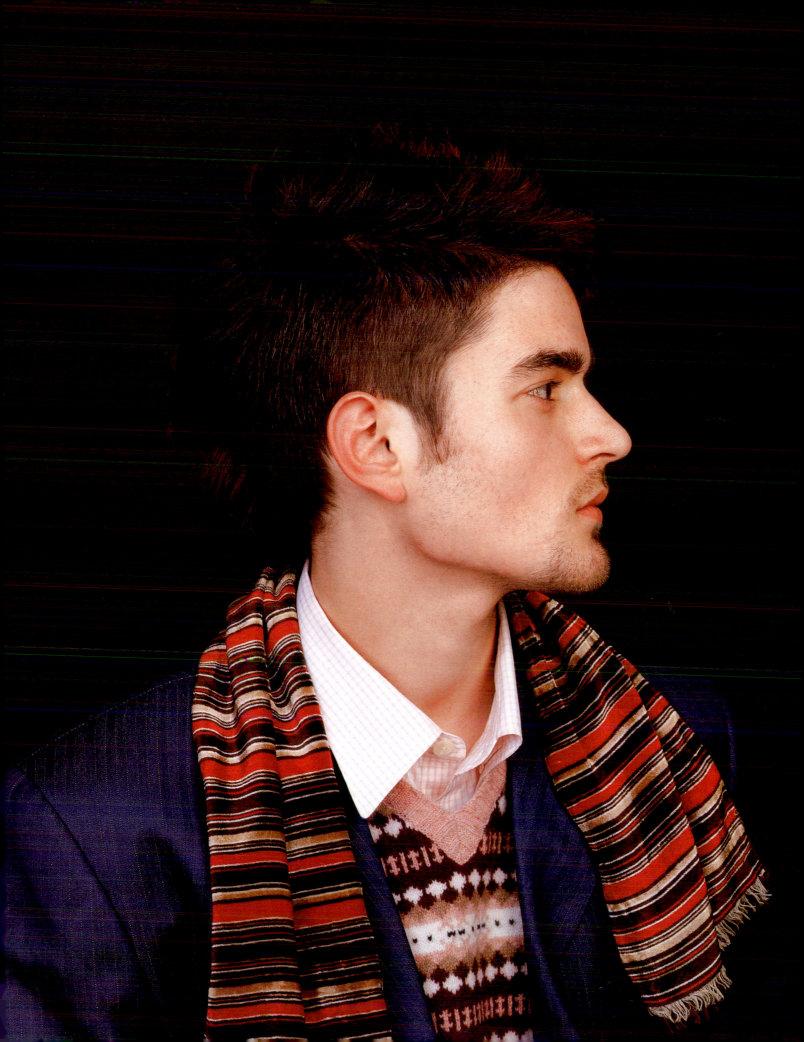

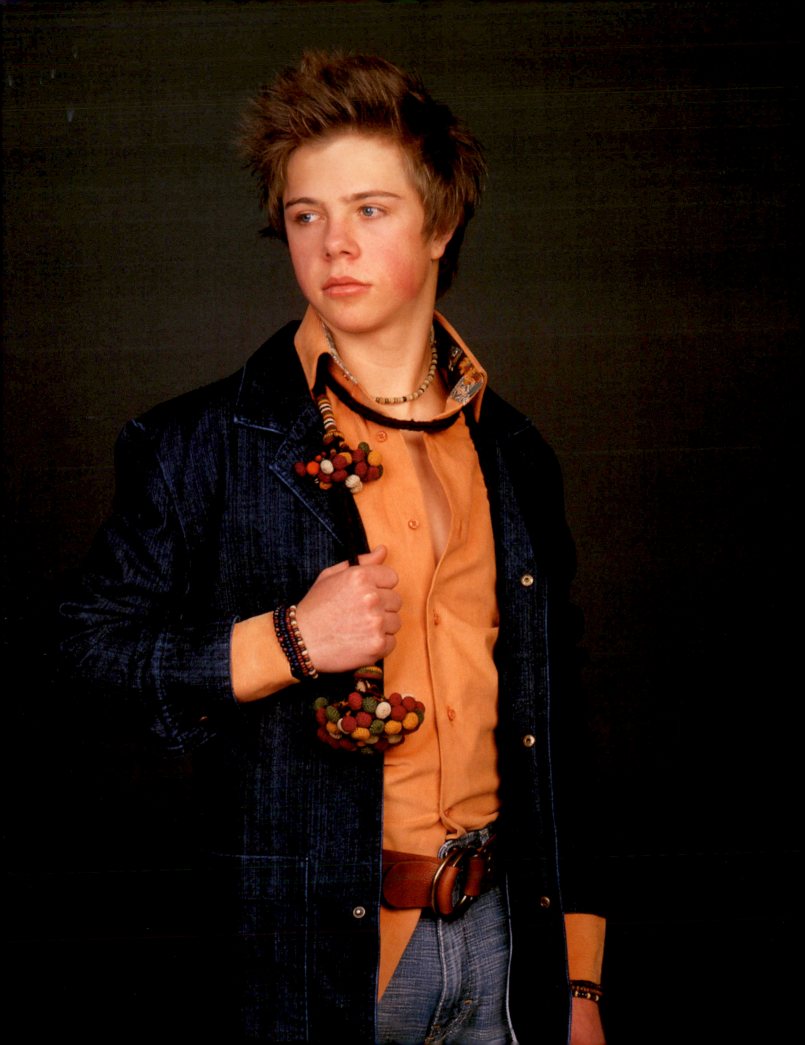

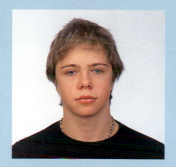

SAM

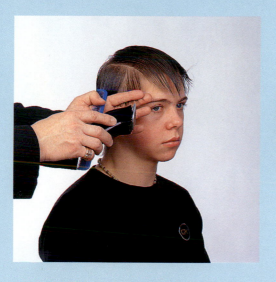

Section off front hair from ear to temple. Take a vertical section from side and use clippers freehand to 'chip into' ends overdirecting the hair forwards.

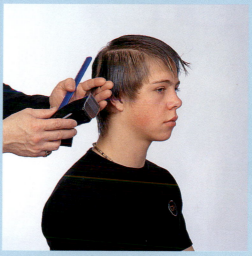

From behind ear, take vertical section and work in the same way, overdirecting the hair forward.

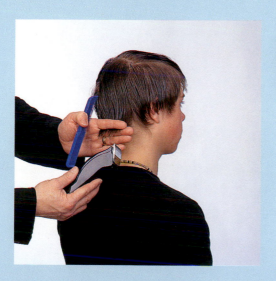

Elevate nape hair and chip into ends at an angle of 45 degrees.

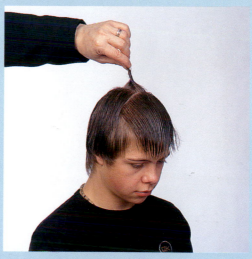

On crown take a 2.5cm section firmly in fingers, twist in a clockwise direction keeping hold of ends.

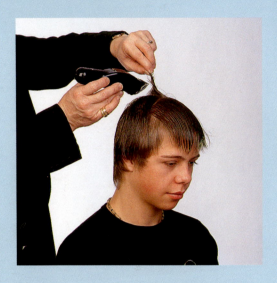

Chip into this twisted section with razor using light strokes.

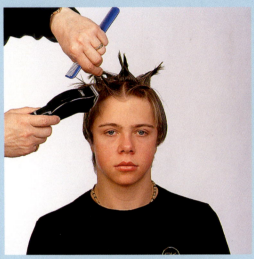

Continue in this manner over entire crown.

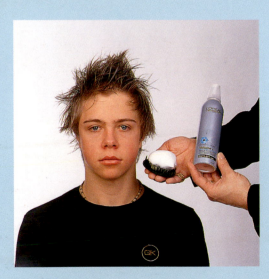

Dispense tecni.art Volume + mousse into palm of hand then distribute evenly through hair to give control and maintain softness.

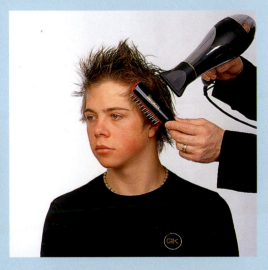

Blow-dry using nozzle attachment and a Classic Styling Brush.

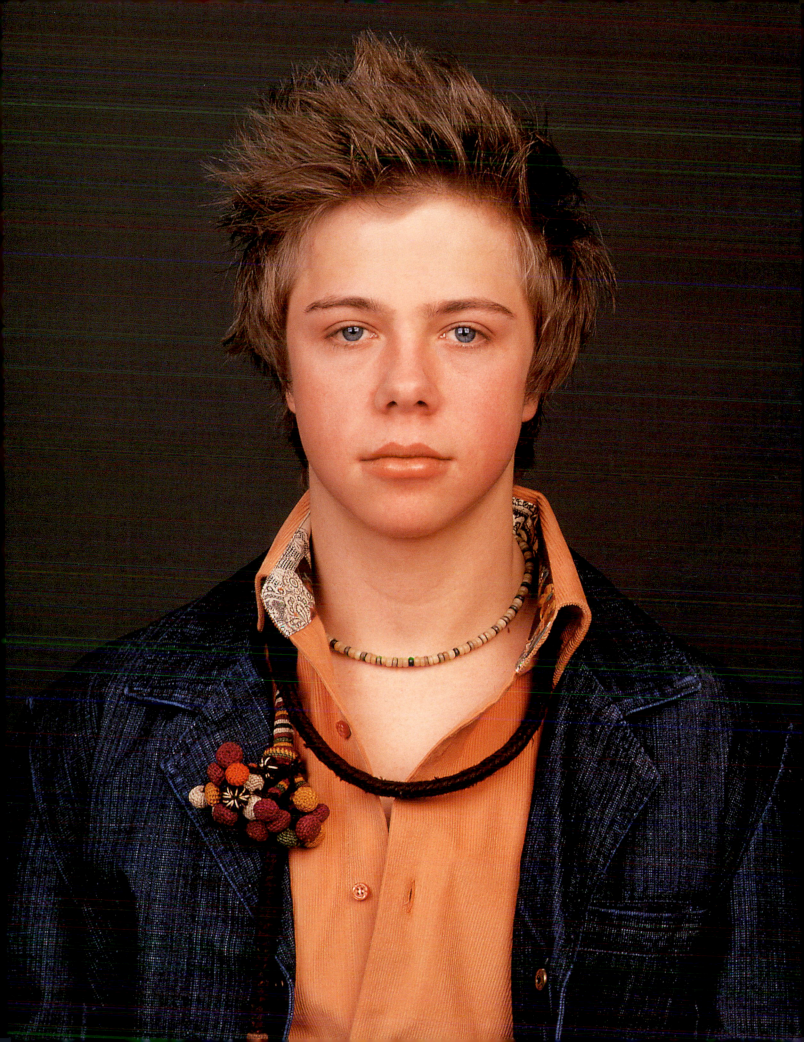

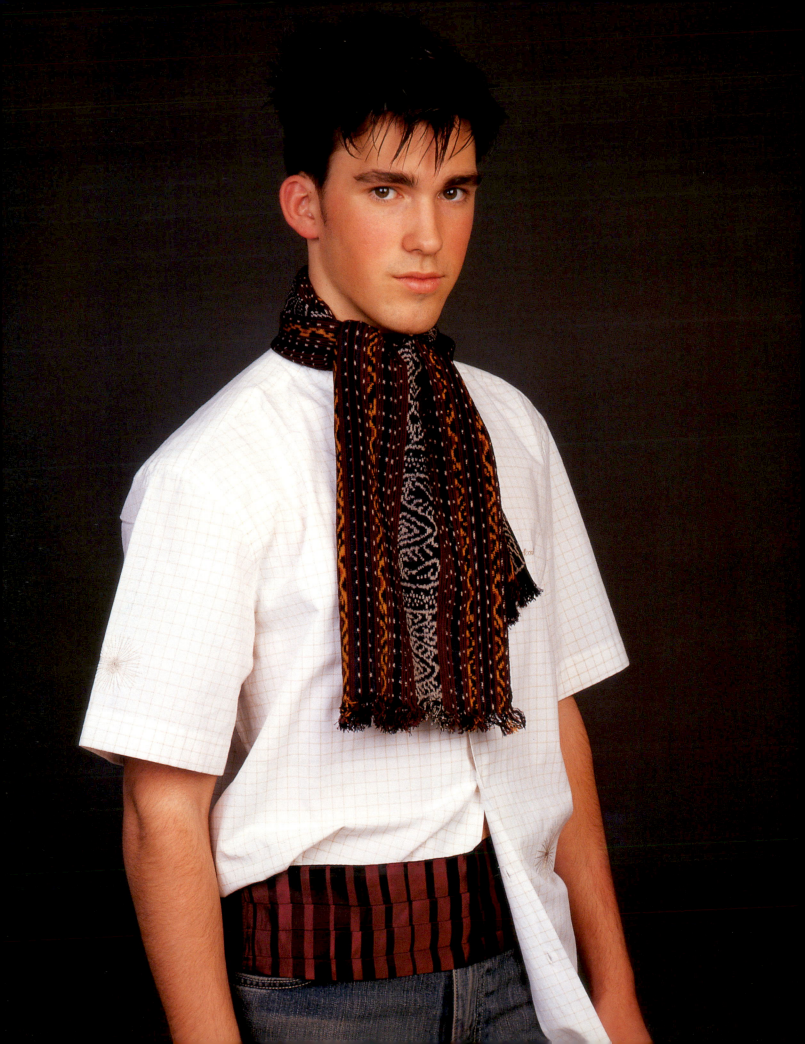

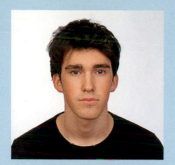

RICHARD

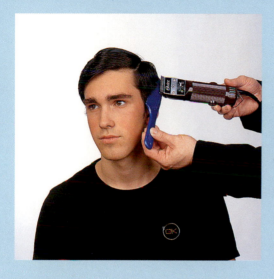

Use clipper over comb to cut side up to temple creating guideline.

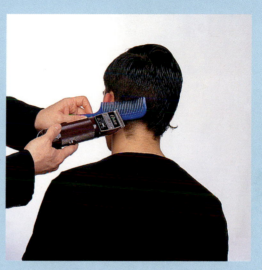

Cut back section using clipper over comb method.

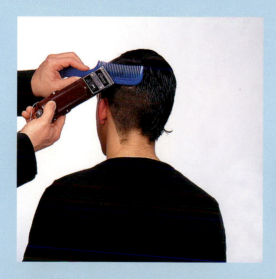

Work up to guideline at back in the same manner.

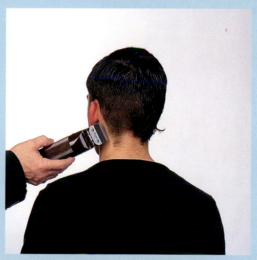

Clean up neck area using clippers.

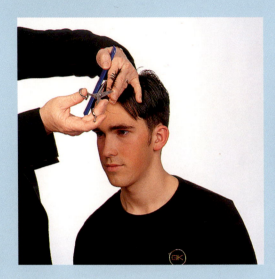

Take a vertical section at front and point cut to remove length and create texture.

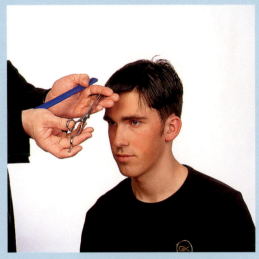

Point cut fringe area.

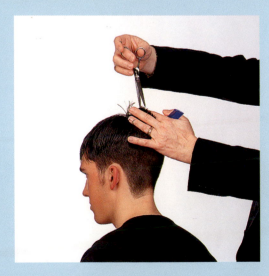

Cut crown area shorter by chipping into ends to give a spiky texture.

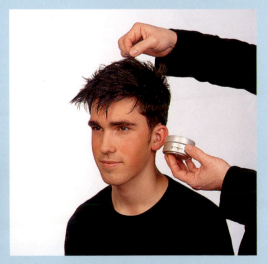

Work tecni.art a-head CLAY through hair to achieve a texturised finish.

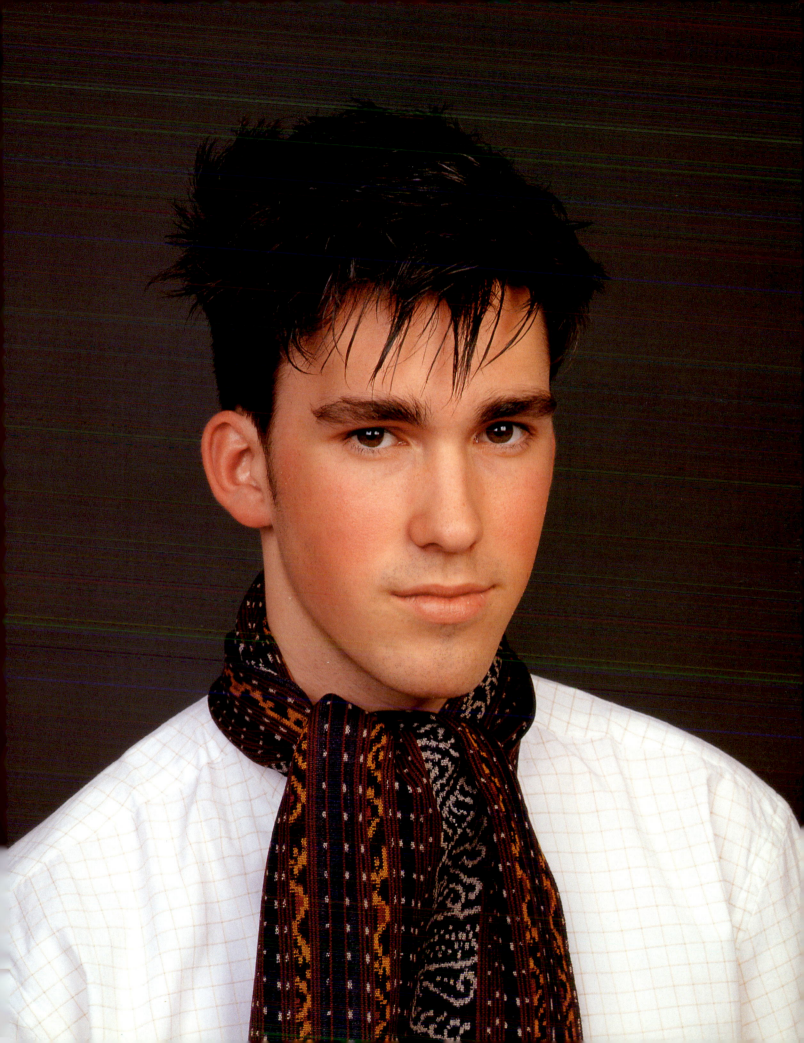

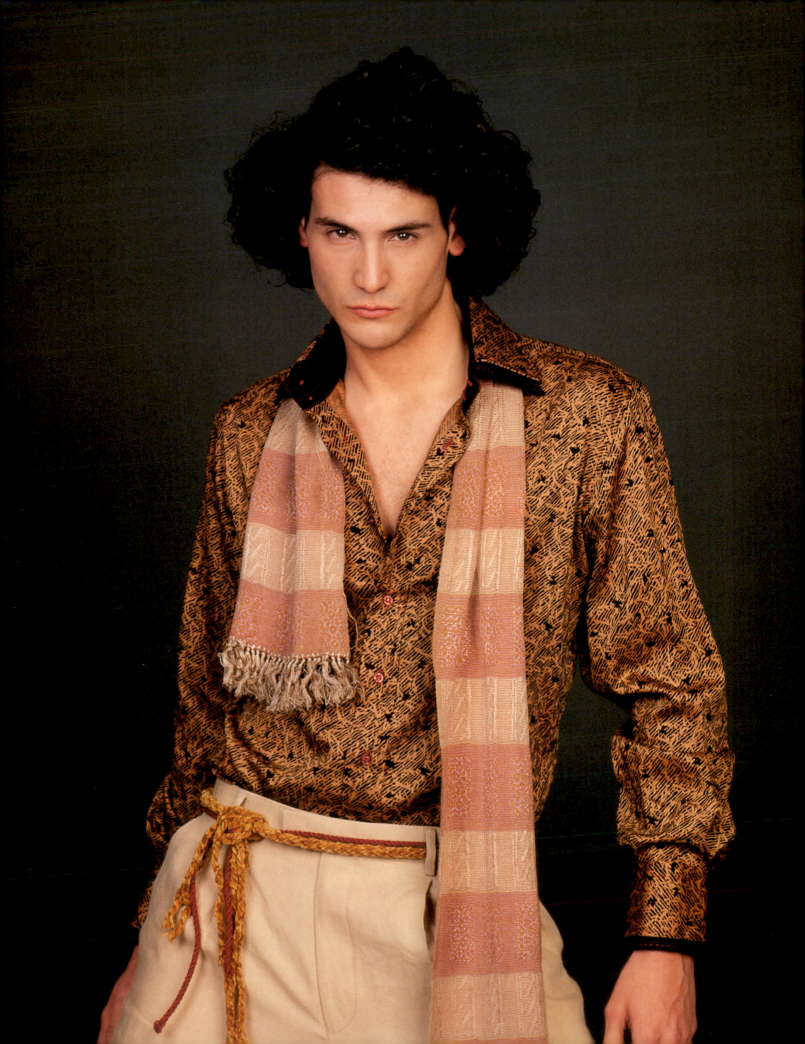

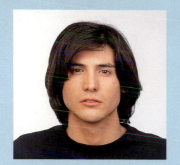

PABLO

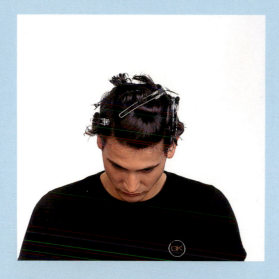

Divide hair into sections as shown.

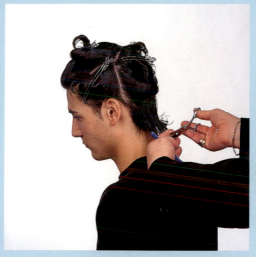

Working on lower nape hair remove 1.5cm of length.

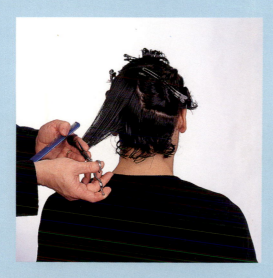

Take next section and remove 1.5cm of length working to first guideline.

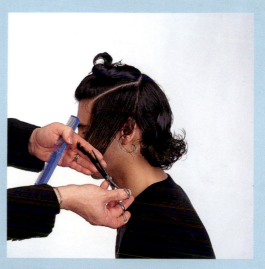

Work on side section overdirecting hair and giving a slightly graduated line. Repeat through other side.

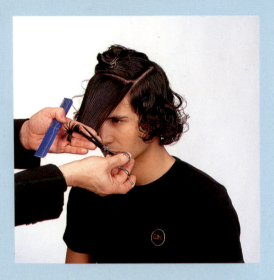

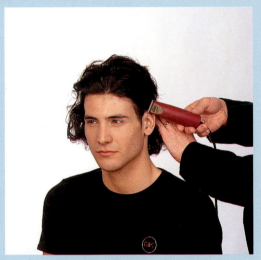

Comb down front section and remove 1.5cm of length. Continue through crown in same manner.

Use finisher clipper to clean up round ears.

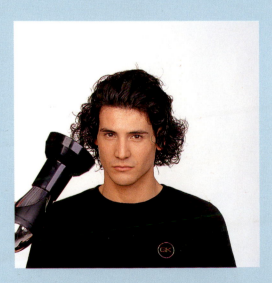

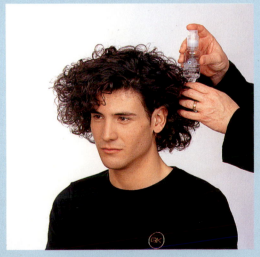

Blow-dry using diffuser attachment, allowing hair to sit in diffuser cup so that it dries gently.

Apply tecni.art Liss control throughout curls to define and smooth.

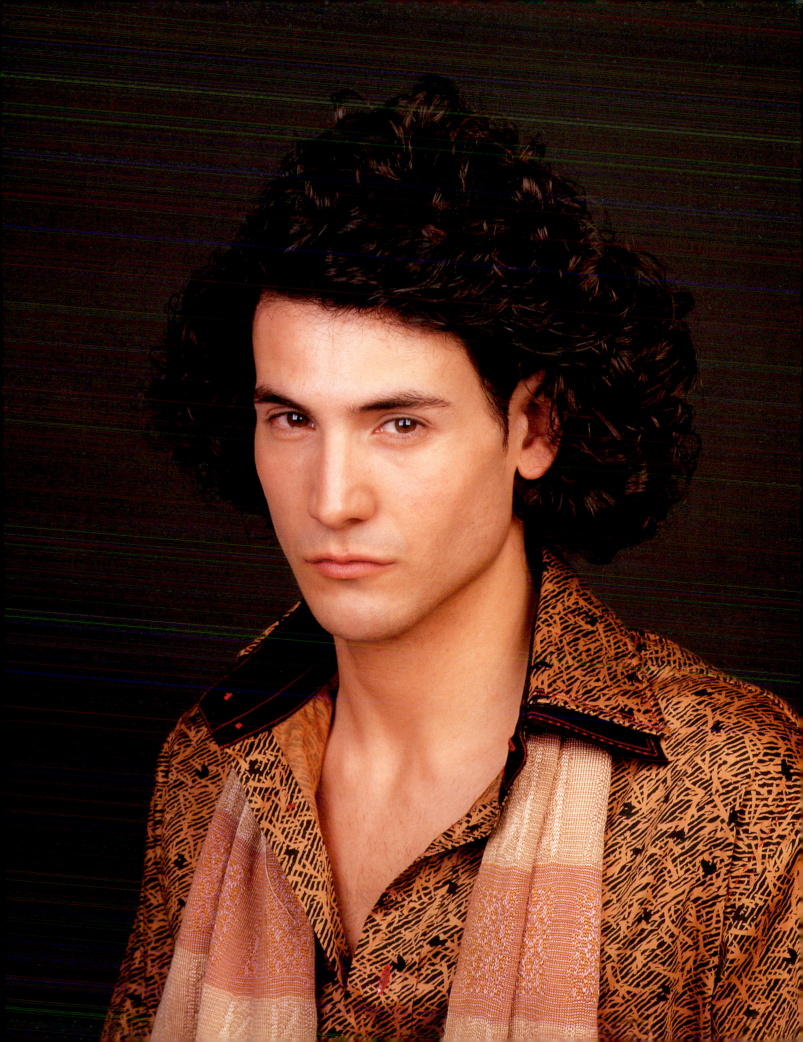

Tools

OF THE TRADE

Backwash and hair care products

The perfect finished look starts at the backwash in the salon. In order to create the best cut and style possible, the correct tools are required and these include products to cleanse and nourish the hair.

Prior to cutting, each client's hair should be analysed by touching and looking at the hair and scalp, and also by asking your client about his hair care regime. How often does he wash his hair? What products does he use? From this analysis and using your expertise in hair, the professional shampoo and conditioner most suited to your clients' hair can be selected.

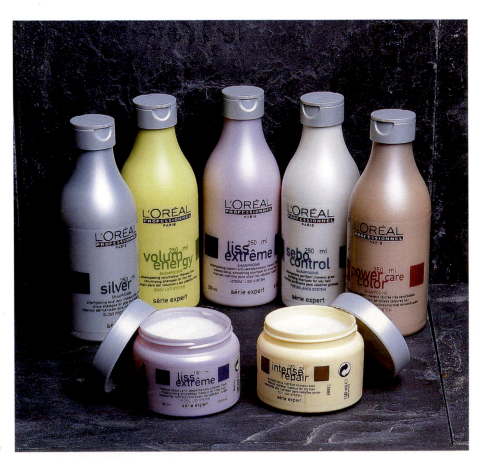

The L'Oréal Professionnel
Série Expert range

KEY INGREDIENTS IN SHAMPOOS AND CONDITIONERS, AND THEIR ACTION ON THE HAIR

Amino Acids like Vitamin E derivatives help maintain the moisture balance of the hair and as such the condition.

Humecants like Pro-Vitamin B5 are used to replace moisture.

UVA and UVB filters can absorb UV light from the sun, which causes hair colour to fade. These filters help to prevent fading and damage to the hair structure.

Surfactants and cleansing agents are designed to cleanse hair, remove impurities and give hair softness. They also help counteract flyaway hair.

Panthenol thickens and enlarges each hair shaft by allowing more moisture and protein to be absorbed into the hair.

Ceramide strengthens the hair fibre by its 'repairing' action depositing within the cuticle layer of the hair fibre, reinforcing the hair structure and helping to repair damaged areas.

TYPES OF CONDITIONERS

Basic conditioners coat the hair shaft with a fine film of oil, smoothing down the cuticle and making hair glossier and easier to manage. These should be used after every shampoo, and combed through for even distribution.

Colour and perm conditioners are for chemically treated hair. After perm conditioners help stabilise hair and are designed to keep bounce in the curl. After colour products add a protective film around porous areas, preventing colour loss and minimising fading.

Conditioning sprays form a protective barrier against the effect of heat styling. They are also good for reducing static on flyaway hair.

Intensive conditioners help hair retain its natural moisture balance, replenishing where necessary. Use if hair is split, dry or frizzy or difficult to manage.

Leave-in conditioners are designed to help retain moisture, reduce static in flyaway hair and add shine. They are good for clients with fine hair as they avoid conditioner overload, which can cause lankness. Ideal for daily use and easy to apply, they provide a protective barrier against the effect of heat-styling.

Restructurants penetrate the cortex, helping to repair and strengthen the inner fibrous structure by rebuilding the linkages. These should be used if hair is lank or limp and has lost its natural elasticity owing to chemical treatments or physical damage.

THE BACKWASH

Applying conditioning treatments at the backwash is an excellent way to relax the client and ensure his hair is in the best condition possible when the leaves the salon. Again it is important to identify the client's hair type as well as his needs. Some clients may have limited time and so an intensive treatment, which offers instant results, would be ideal. Others may want to feel pampered and will have time for a luxurious full head massage.

The backwash also represents the perfect opportunity to offer the clients hints and tips about how to care for their hair at home. Clients appreciate your expert recommendations about products they can take home with them to ensure the result they get in the salon can be recreated at home. By taking time to prescribe and use the correct shampoo and conditioner you ensure that you get the best possible overall result.

Clippers

Clippers are not just for crew cuts. They form a useful companion to scissors and can be used for tapering, trimming, thinning, feathering, undercutting, channelling and fringing. They are also ideal for cutting Afro hair and can be used to create strong outline shapes on the hairline, or used to carry out a complete haircut.

HOW THEY WORK

The principle is of one fixed and one moving blade. Each blade has sharp teeth and the action of the moving blade cuts the hair. It can be likened to several pairs of scissors being used simultaneously – as many as 14,400 cutting strokes per minute can be made with some types of electric clipper.

The type of clipper you choose depends on whether you need just a general-purpose tool for lining out and trimming neck and side-burns, or if you prefer to incorporate clipper techniques into most of your hair cuts. If so a heavy duty pair would be your best choice.

Electric clippers are operated by an electric motor in the body of the clipper. When switched on, one blade constantly moves across the other. Magnetic motors are on direct drive, giving high-speed movements. Clippers can run directly from the mains electricity, or be cordless (rechargeable). Adjusting the blades ($\frac{1}{20}$mm for the closest to 3mm for the longest alters the closeness of the cut).

A variety of comb attachments can be used on clippers and these can be graded, 1,2,3 and 4 or $\frac{1}{16}$", $\frac{1}{8}$", $\frac{1}{4}$", $\frac{3}{8}$", $\frac{1}{2}$" and 1". Most clippers also come with a blending guide.

Cordless or rechargeable trimmers are suitable for outlining, trimming and detail work, for cleaning-up hair lines, neck lines, side-burns, moustaches and beards. They give convenient freedom of movement and most can be used for up to 60 minutes on one charge.

POINTS TO NOTE

When choosing a clipper check the weight, balance, vibration and noise factor in use. Some clippers are contoured to fit hands. Detachable blades make sterilising easy and more efficient. Buy from a reputable supplier who offers a guarantee and after sales service facilities.

Clipper cuts have enjoyed various periods of popularity. Initially worn by German forces during the First World War, the look was adopted by American seamen – hence the name, Crew Cut. Initially the regulation length was one inch on top, but in the mid-Twenties this was increased to two inches.

It wasn't until 1948 that the Marine Corps decreed that the two-inch haircut was an ugly length. It was decided that, from that time, officers and enlisted men should wear their hair neatly and closely trimmed. Hair was to be clipped at the edges of the sides and the back had to be trimmed to present an evenly graduated appearance, not over three inches in length. Since that time, the closely-shaven head has always had military overtones.

CLIPPER CARE

- Blades should be aligned following manufacturers' instructions.
- Clipper blades must be kept well-oiled with an oil specifically designed for this purpose. Most manufacturers' suggest oiling before and after each cut and many traditional barbers oil their clippers half way through a cut as well. Most blades that are returned to manufacturers' as 'blunt' merely haven't been oiled properly.
- Do not use clippers with broken teeth as this can result in dragging the hair and cutting the skin.
- Always use a blade guard when clippers are not in use.
- Check manufacturers' advice about sterilising your clippers. It is not advisable to take electric clippers apart, although some clipper heads are removable for cleaning.
- If clippers pull hair, try cleaning and adjusting them.
- Always return to manufacturer or supplier for repairs.

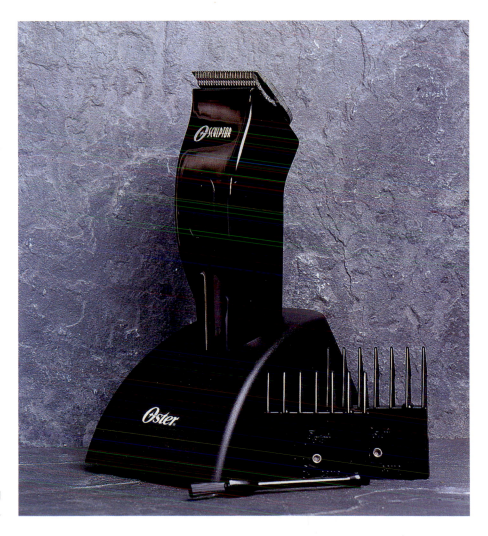

Choose a professional clipper and check the weight and balance.

Brushes and Combs

Brushes are available in many different shapes and sizes to suit all hair types and grooming needs. They help remove tangles, loosen dead skin cells and dirt and encourage the cuticles to lie flat, thus reflecting light and giving hair a high gloss finish. Brushing also stimulates the blood and lymph supply to the hair follicles and helps promote healthy hair growth.

A brushes' most important role is that of styling as they allow you to smooth, curl, straighten, lift and add volume to hair quickly and easily.

As we use different shampoos and conditioners to suit hair types and textures we also need different brushes to achieve various finishes. In fact, no self-respecting hairdresser has less than a full wardrobe of brushes to choose from.

BRUSHES

Classic styling
Half-round brushes with smooth round ended nylon quills set into an anti-static natural rubber pad.
Ideal for   All lengths and types of hair.
Use to   Smooth, shape and polish the hair.

Curling
Round brushes with flexible nylon or bristle set into plastic or wooden handles. Available in a variety of diameters – the smaller the barrel, the tighter the curl. Some designs have bristles set into a metal barrel which retains hairdryer heat thus reducing drying time.
Ideal for   Short, mid-length or long wavy or curly hair.
Use to   Curl and smooth short hair or smooth and straighten longer hair. Ideal for flicking hair under or out.

Grooming
Oval shaped brushes with pure natural bristle or bristle/nylon mix set into an air-cushioned rubber pad.
Ideal for   Polishing all lengths of fine to normal hair and for removing loose hairs.
Use to   Smooth and style hair into shape. The bristles polish the hair, spreading the natural oils down the shaft to give a brilliant shine. Available in small, medium and large sizes the brushes are an investment purchase for hairdressers and clients.

Paddle
Flat brushes with ball-tipped nylon pins set in a soft rubber air cushion base. The staggered pin pattern means that the brush glides through the hair without dragging or stretching.
Ideal for   All types and lengths of hair including very long locks.
Use to   Detangle hair after shampooing and conditioning. Lift and straighten hair when blow drying or simply for grooming.

Vent
Lightweight, vented brushes with widely spaced pins that allow warm air to circulate directly at root level accelerating the blow-drying process.
Ideal for   All lengths and types of hair.
Use to   Detangle and gently blow-dry hair smooth, create texture and movement. Used by session hairdressers to get fast and effective results.

Volumising Half-round brushes with round-ended widely spaced nylon pins set into an anti-static natural rubber pad.
Ideal for All hair types including detangling thicker hair and styling curls.
Use to Add volume and smooth hair whilst blow-drying.

COMBS

Combs also come in a wide variety of shapes and sizes and each design has a specific function. It is important to always use combs with round ended pins to protect the hair and scalp from damage.

Cutting comb has both narrow and widely spaced teeth. Used for cutting and styling.
Detangling comb has wide-spaced teeth to gently separate and detangle all hair lengths and types.
Fantail comb has wide-spaced teeth to separate thick hair for styling. The fantail ends lifts and teases the hair.
Grooming comb has medium spaced teeth suitable for all hair textures.
Styling comb combines a narrow tooth style to groom finer hair and a wide tooth shorter end for lift and to tease the hair.
Tail comb has a pointed end for sectioning and lifting and narrow teeth at the other end for styling.

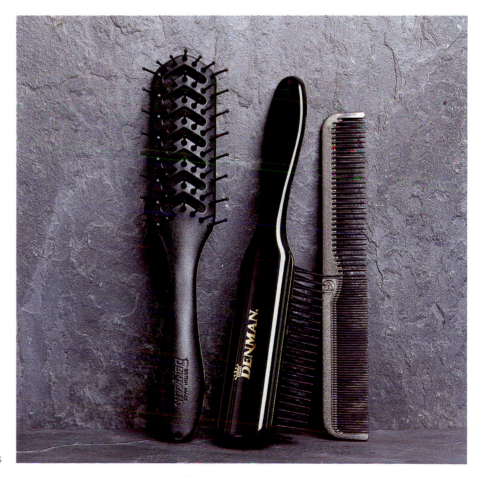

Use professional brushes and combs

Styling products

Hair and fashion have always been linked, but hair is increasingly being considered as much a fashion accessory as make-up or jewellery. Both the hairdresser and client can use styling products to their best advantage to give their own unique feel to any hairstyle and make this accessory truly their own. Whether it's a sleek style straight from the catwalk or the just-out-of-bed look you are looking to achieve, professional products offer all you need for individual self-expression.

Firm Hold Hairspray	Forms an invisible film over hair. Ingredients include resins for hold, proteins to maintain strength and protective emollients to increase pliability and shine.
Variants	From light and flexible to super-strong hold.
Use	Holding, shaping and adding shine.
Gel	Varies in consistency and contains water-soluble ingredients to allow flexibility. Some are oil-based emulsions where microscopic particles of oil give a non-greasy feel, while others contain alcohol, which increases the drying properties.
Variants	Wet look, luminising, fixing
Use	Accentuating shorter styles, dressing, texturising, slicking and moulding.
Mousse	Formulated with polymers and conditioning agents in a mixture of water and alcohol, and dispensed in the form of foam. Mousse provides natural, flexible hold and body, in much the same way as traditional setting/styling lotions.
Variants	Available in different strengths according to the holding power required.
Use	Blow-drying, scrunching, diffuser-drying and finger-drying.
Wax	A solid substance in a pot, this product is made from waxes such as carnauba, ceresin or ozokerite, softened with other ingredients such as mineral oil and lanolin to make it pliable. Some contain vegetable wax and oil to give added gloss and sheen. Other variants are foaming and water–soluble and leave no residue. Soft and hard variants are available.
Variants	Pomade, cream, clay, gum
Use	Dressing, controlling frizz and static, slicking back, defining, moulding and building body. Firm-hold types can be used to create more sculptured styles.
Water Soluble Serum	Made from oils or silicones designed to improve shine and softness by forming a microscopic film on the hair surface. A glossing product which also contains polymers to smooth the cuticle, this works by enrobing it with a protective film and, depending on the product, UV filters. Formulations can vary from light and silky, to heavier, again depending on the desired final look.
Variants	Glosser, polisher.
Use	Improves feel, combating static, de-frizzing, adding shine and gloss.

Many hairdressers, particularly session stylists, like to personalise their hairstyling creations by combining different products in imaginative ways to achieve the result they desire. A favourite 'trick of the trade' is to mix a professional leave-in conditioner with a firm gel which will give a controlled hold that is also soft and pliable. Recently L'Oréal Professionnel's tecniart styling range has introduced a new product to promote this mixing technique in Fix boost, tecni.art's first ever professional styling concentrate. An easy-to-apply 'booster' gel, it is designed to offer the user a chance to personalise their existing favourite styling products with just the right hold for them. For example, your favourite serum, you love the product but you wish the hold was just a little stronger ... just mix in several drops of Fix boost with your serum, apply as normal and you've just created your very own personalised look. Mixing products together to create your own variant is not limited to Fix boost and serums; any good professional styling range will allow this personalisation ... so have fun and mix it up in style!!

Setting or fixing lotions	Provide a high degree of hold and often contain alcohol so they are quick drying. A well-formulated lotion should also contain anti-static ingredients to prevent hair becoming flyaway as the style is brushed through. That, along with its body-adding qualities, makes setting lotion ideal for fine hair and whole-head application. These lotions contain plastic resins and polymers, dissolved in a mixture of alcohol and water, leaving a film or resin on hair when the liquids have evaporated. Lotions come in different formulae designed to give gentle, normal or maximum hold. There are variations for dry/coloured or sensitised hair, others to give volume and additional shine. These days, formulations have a high concentration of flexible resins and are packed in bottles, sprays and pumps. They also provide protection against heat styling.
Variants	Sculpting spray, moulding mist, blow-dry lotion.
Use	Setting, scrunching, blow-drying and natural drying.

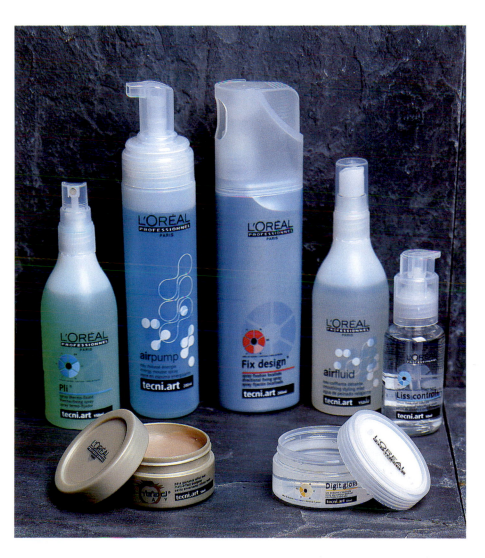

L'Oréal Professionnel tecni-art

Style

GALLERY

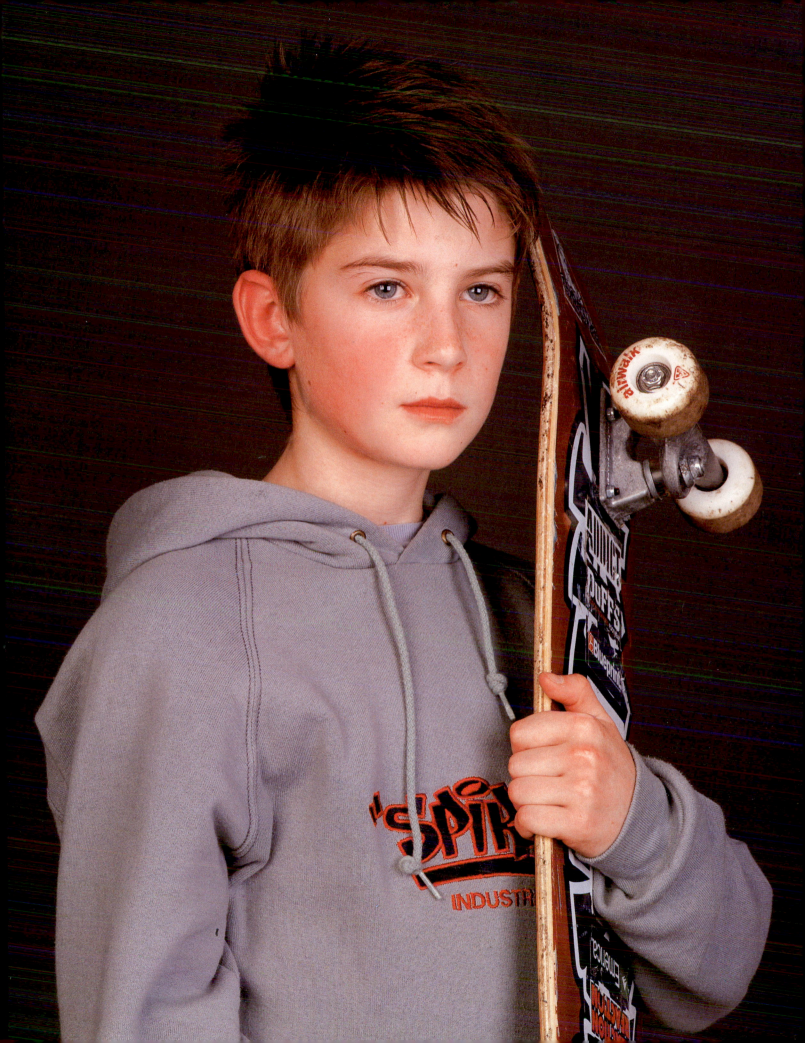

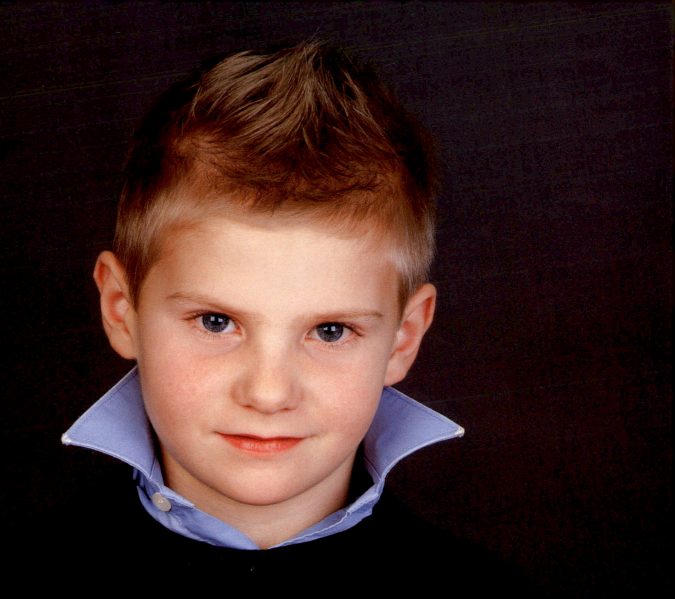

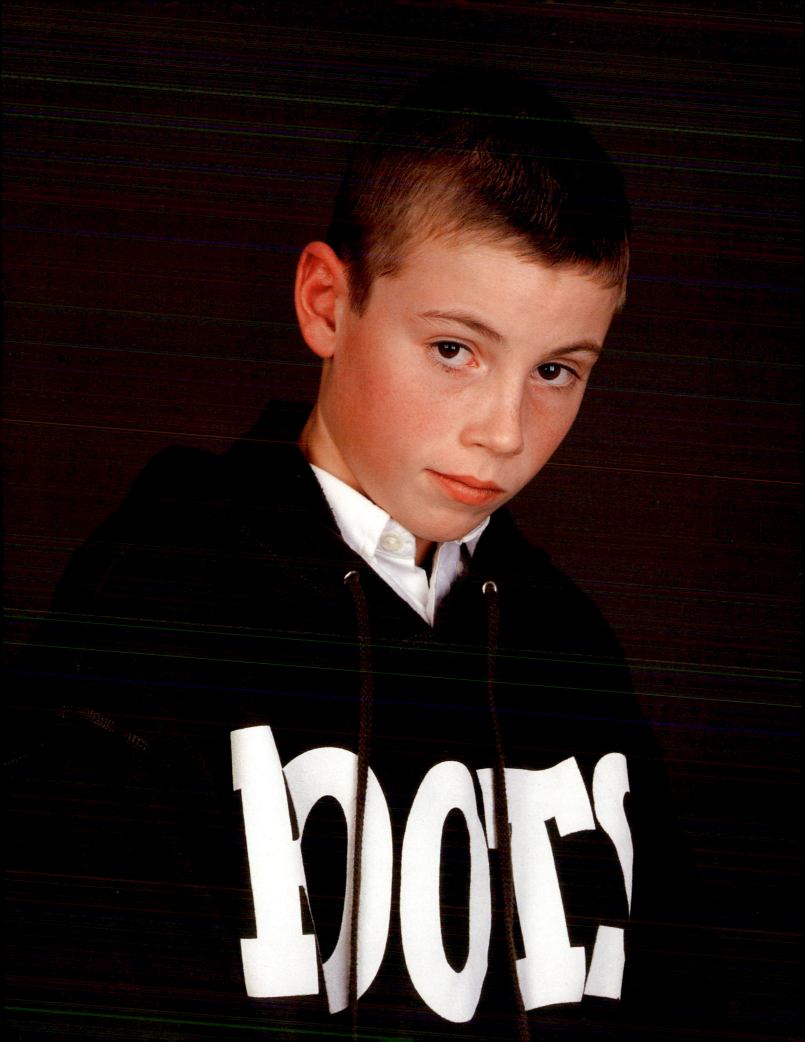

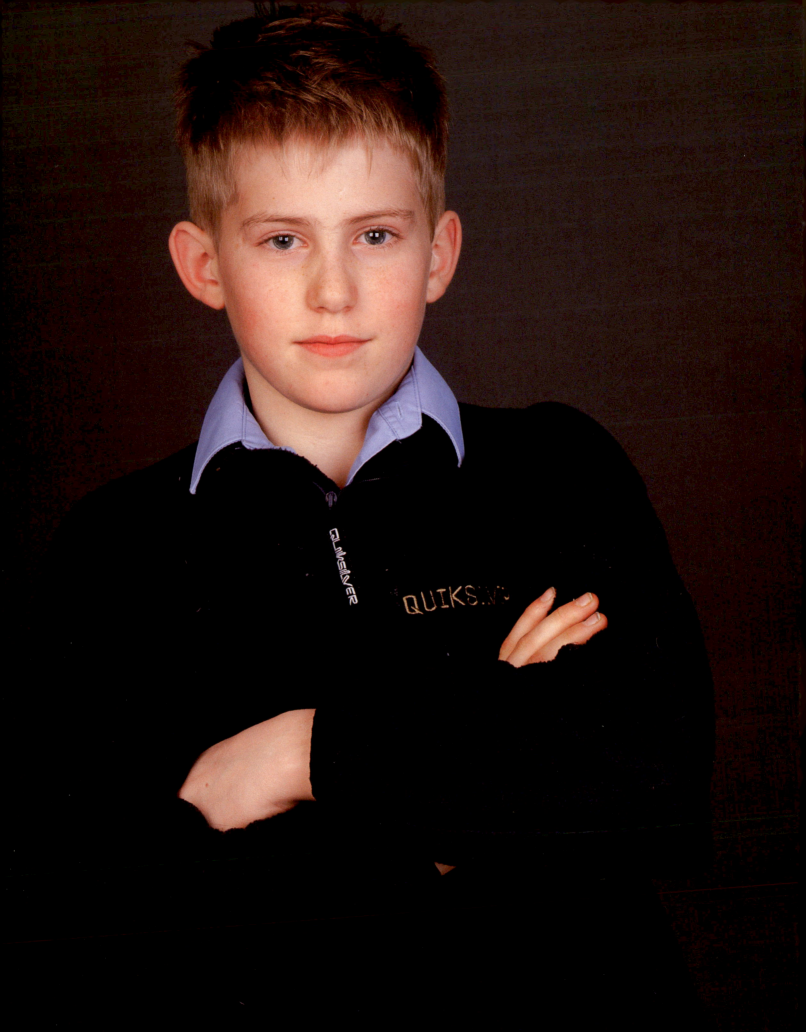

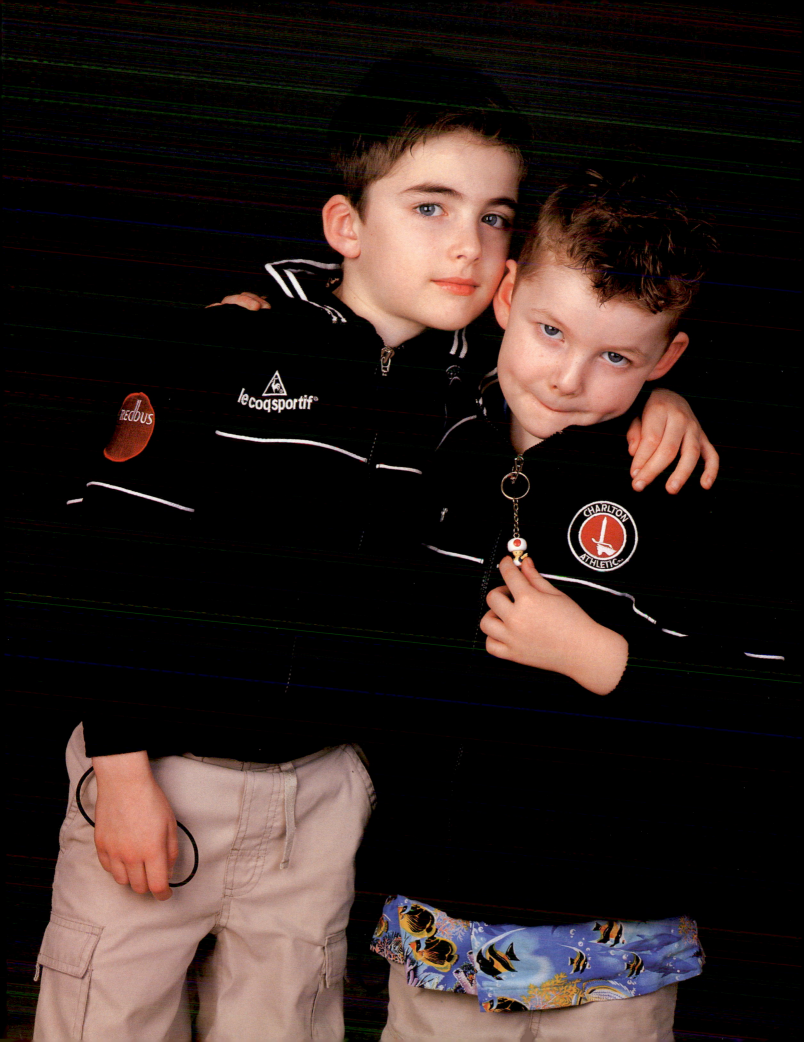

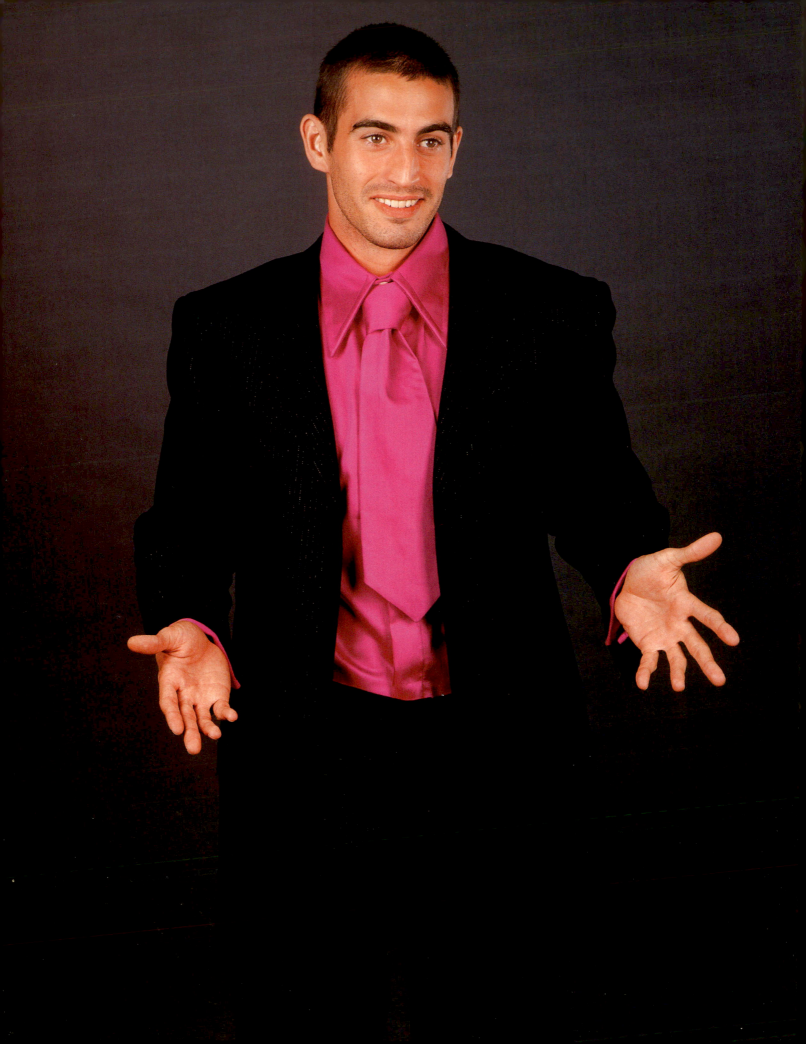

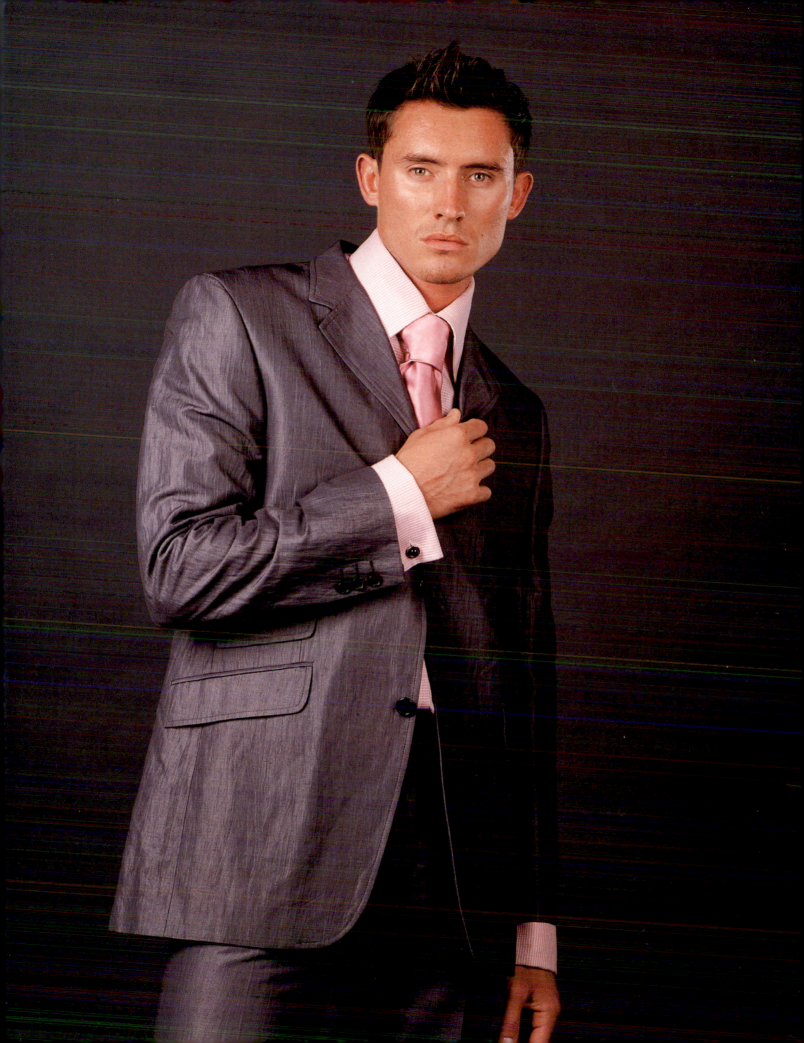

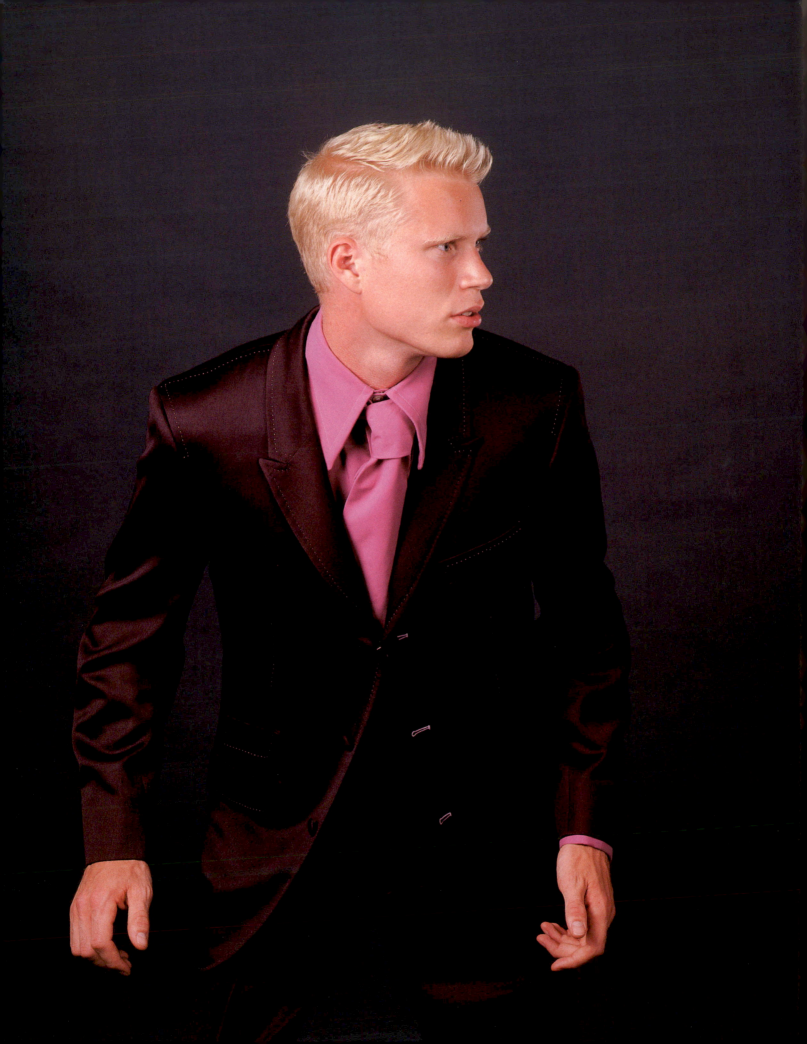

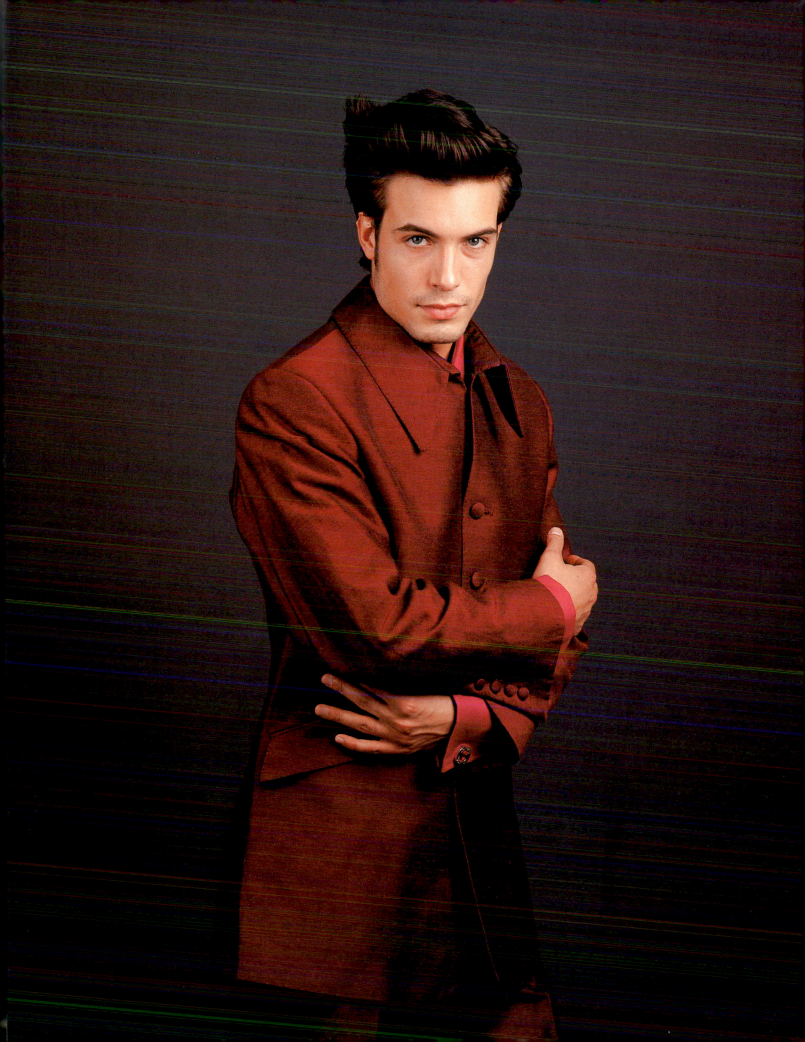

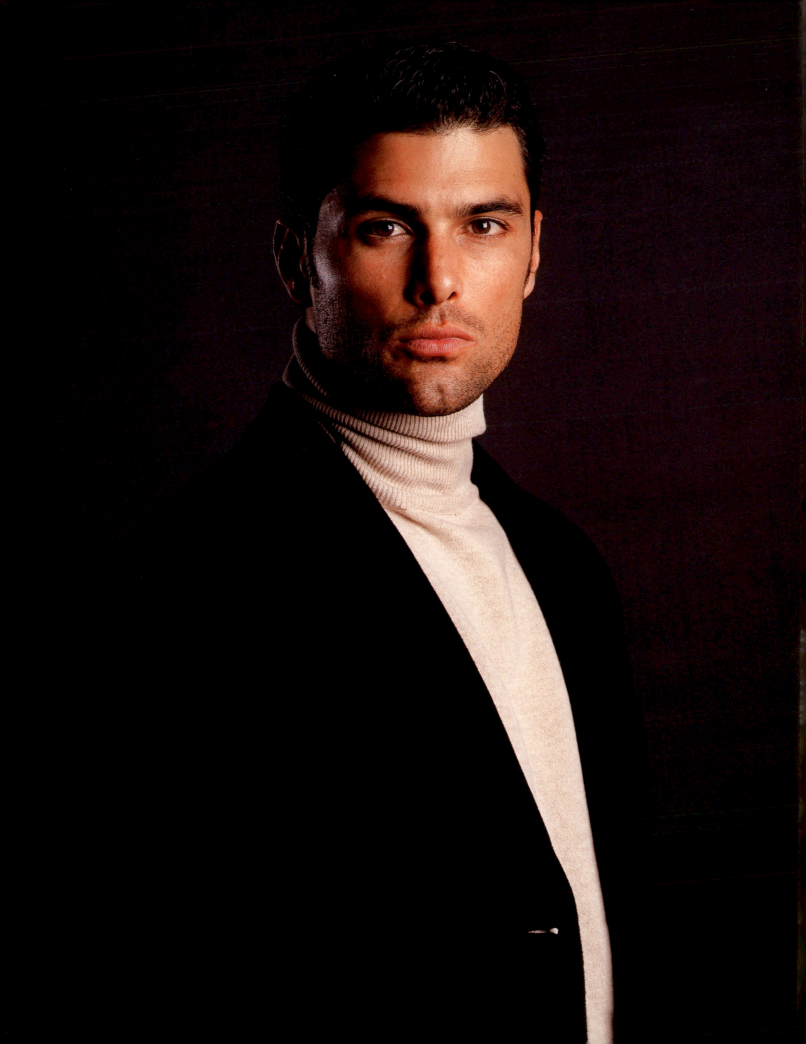

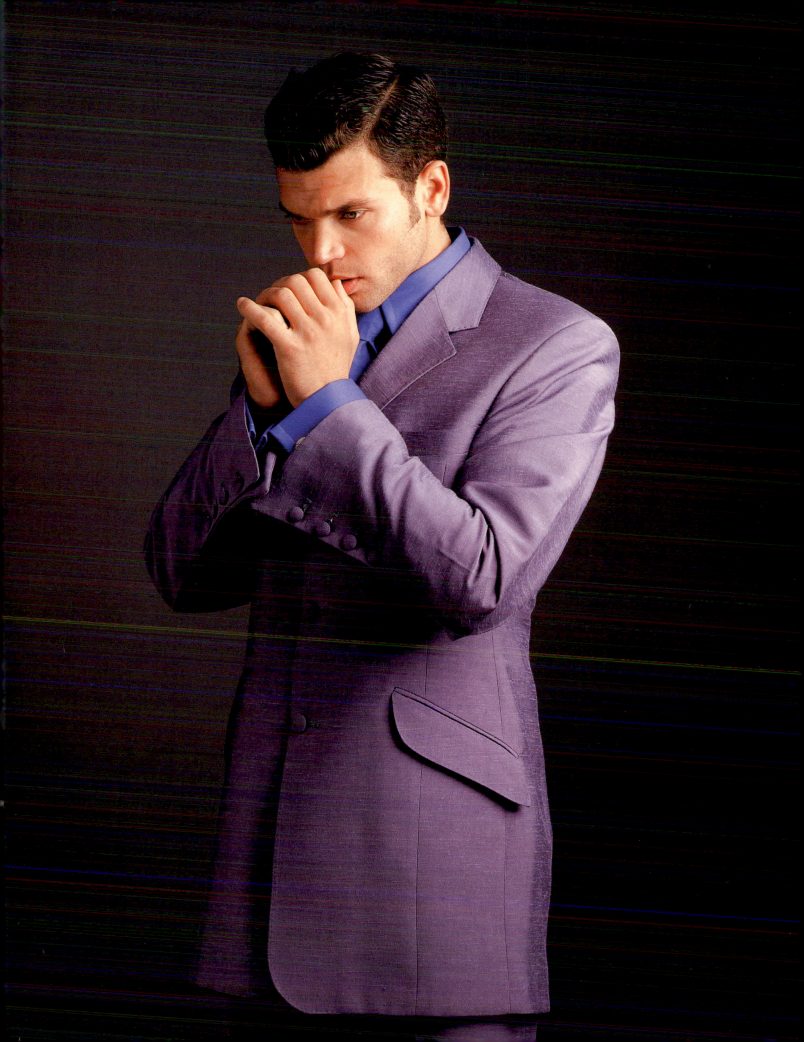

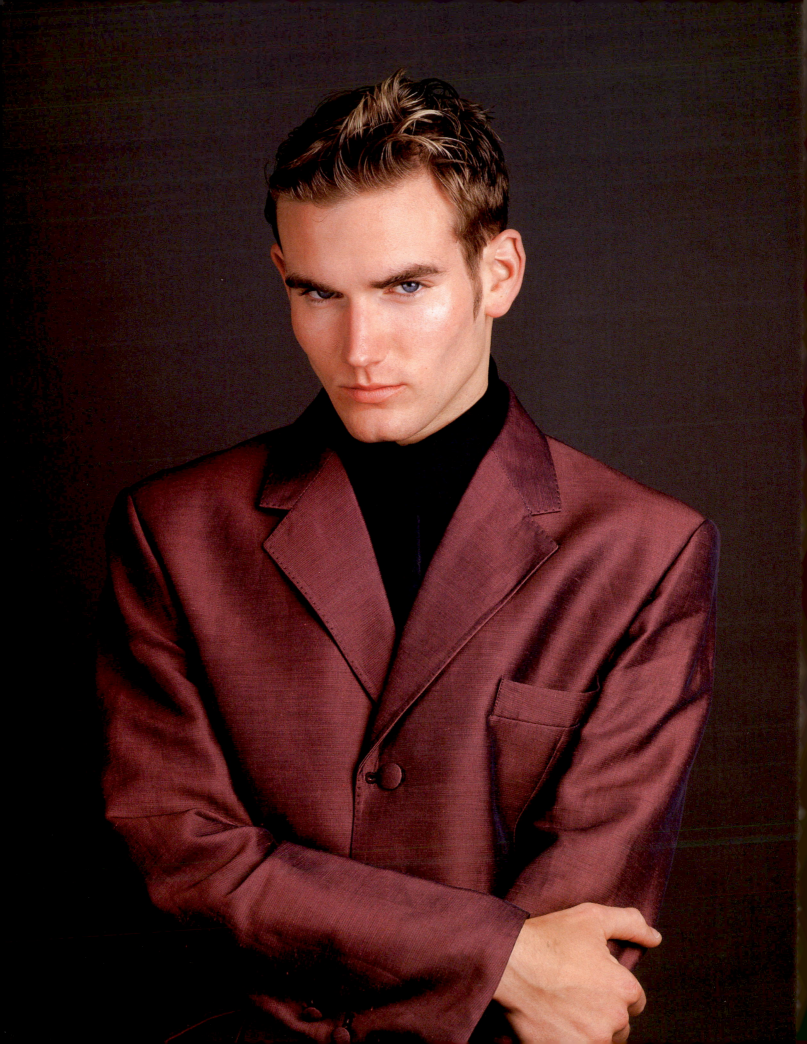

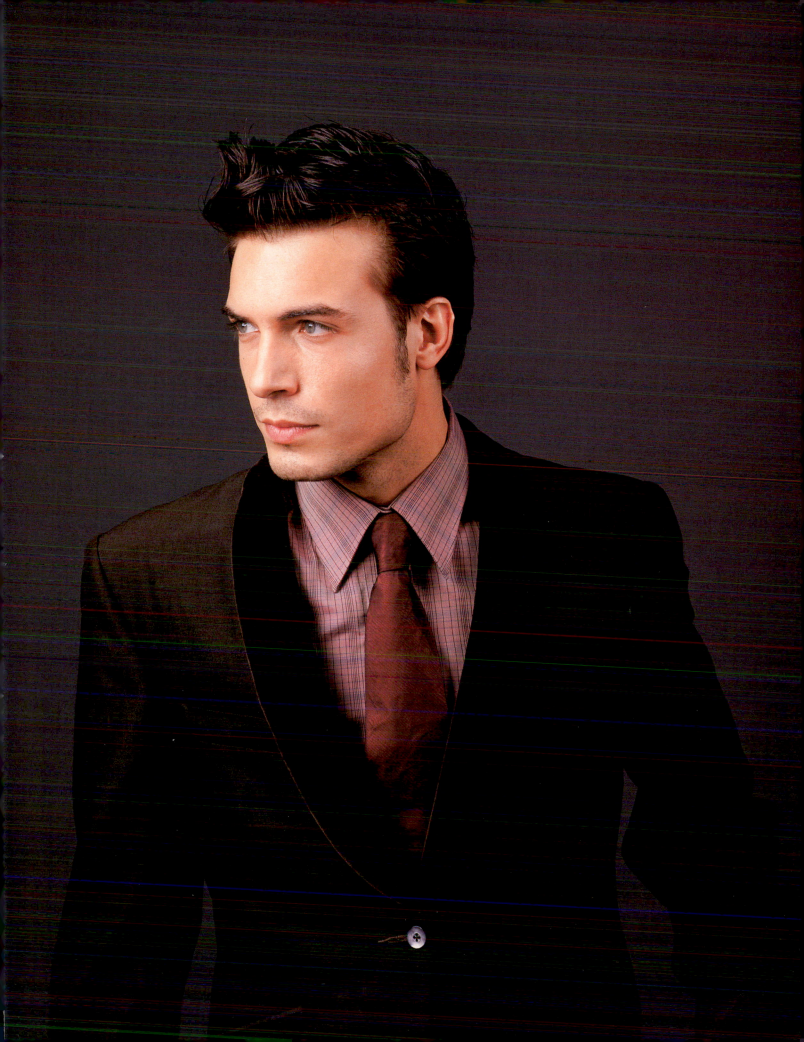

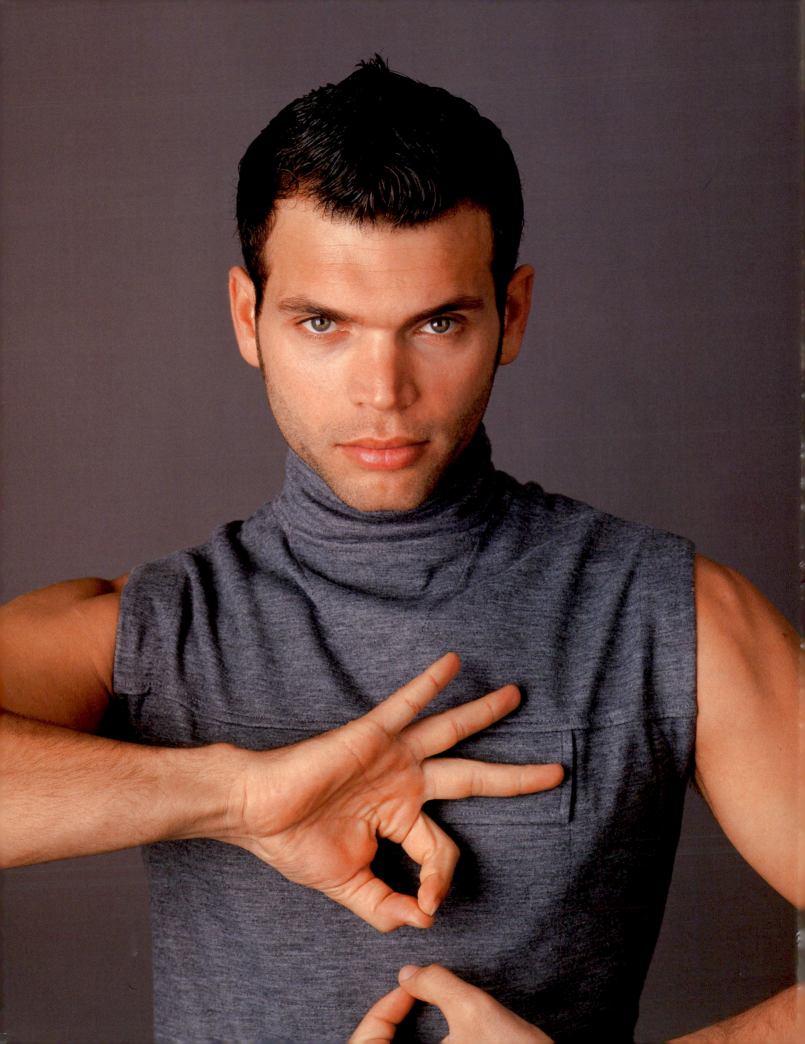

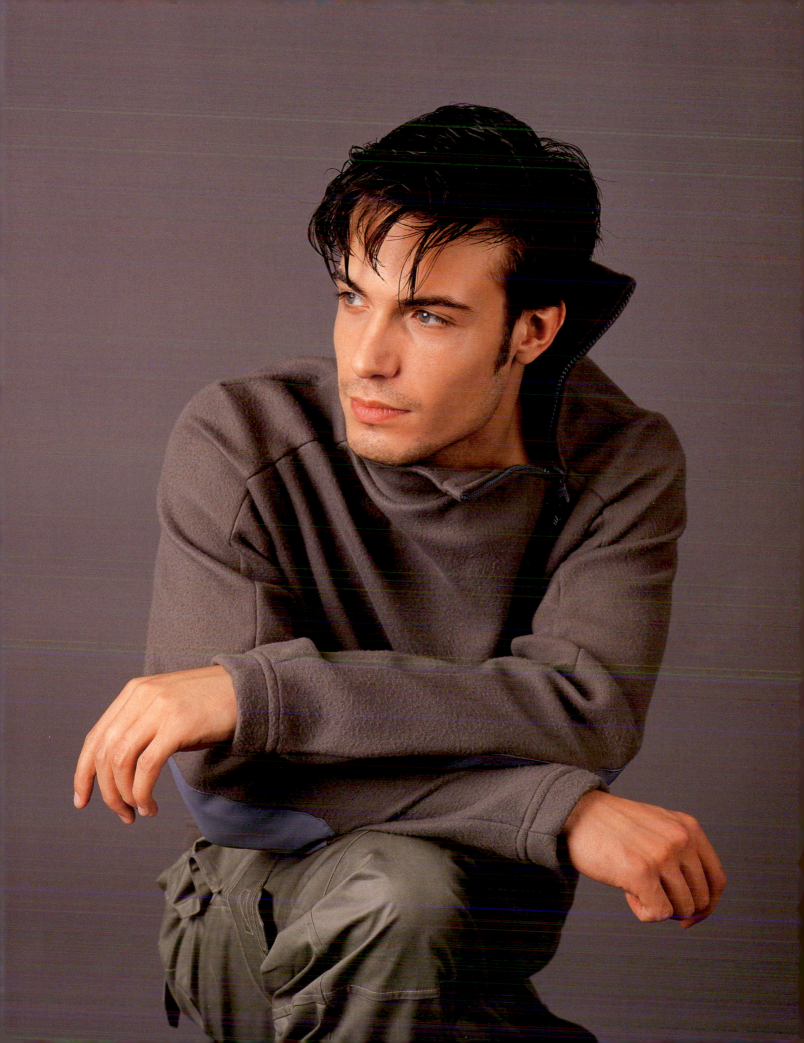

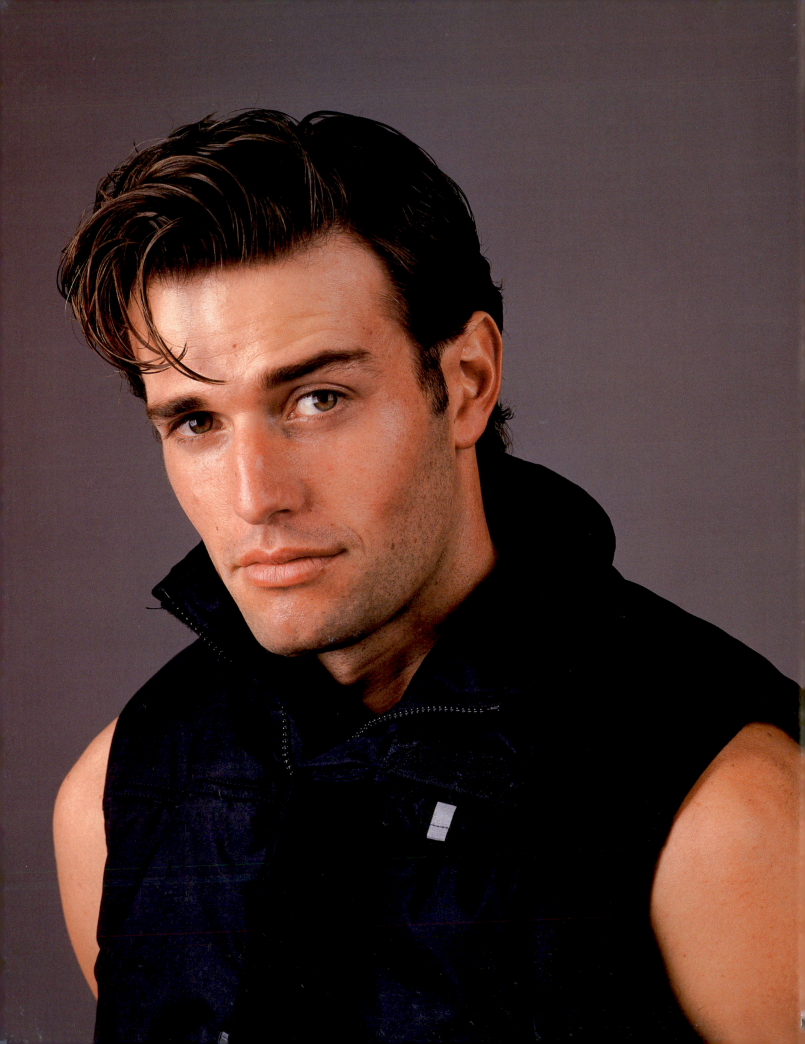

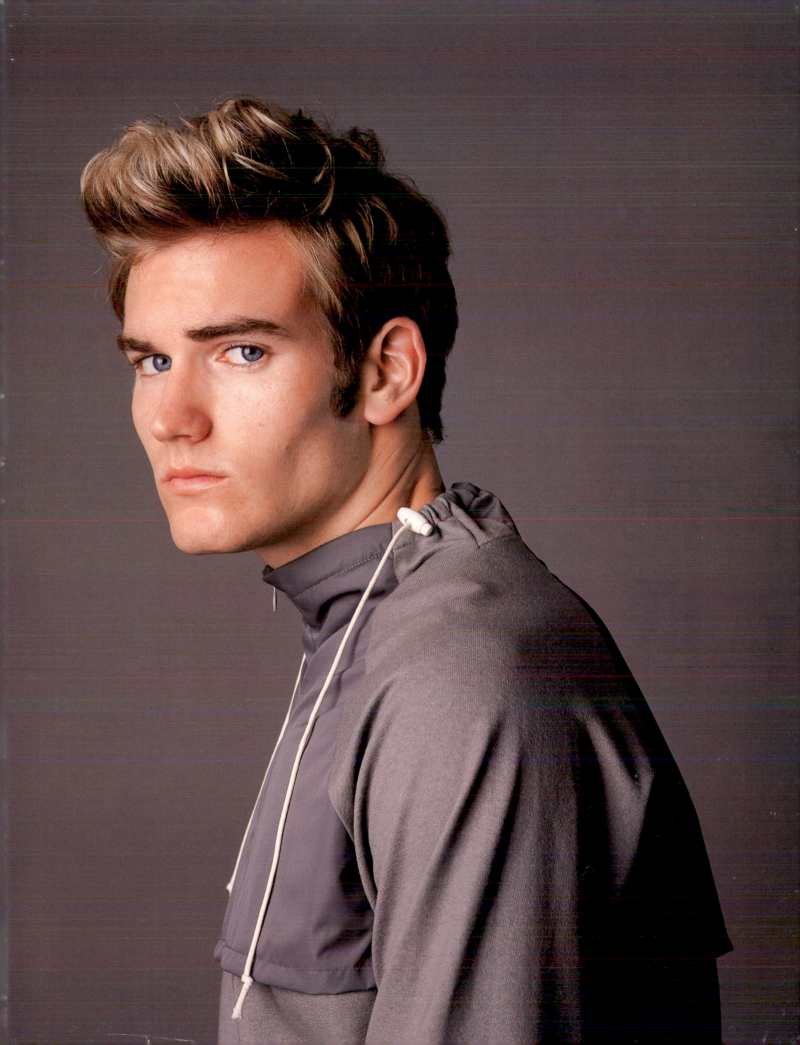

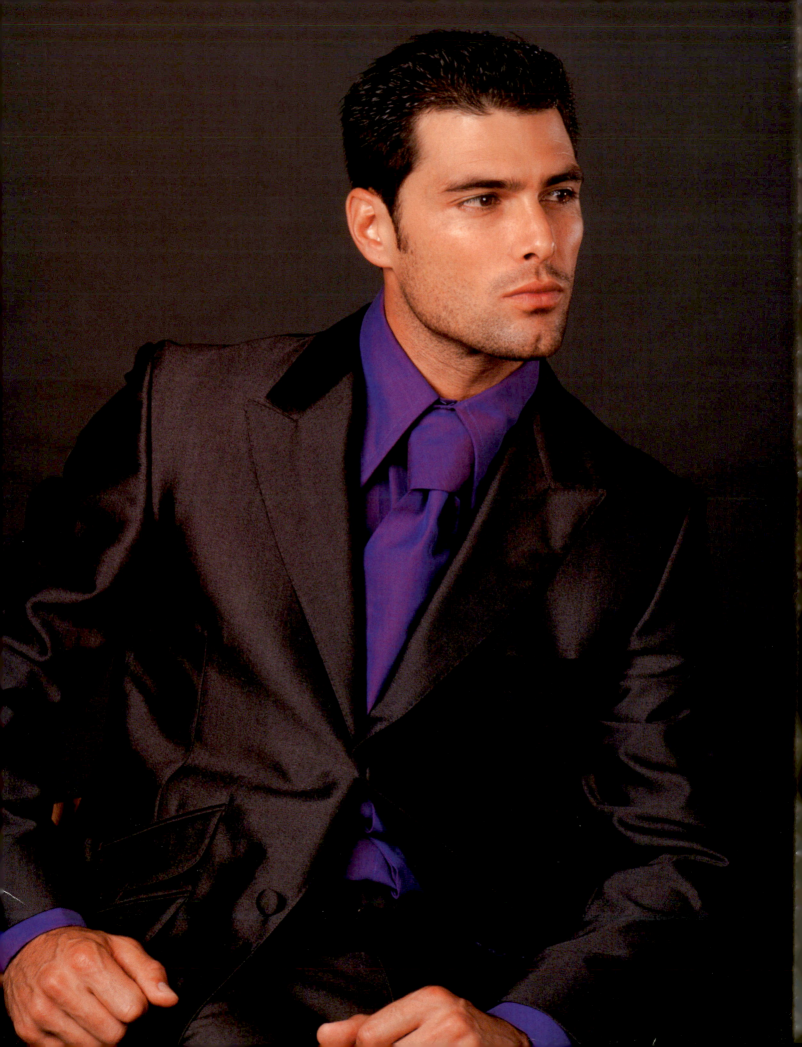

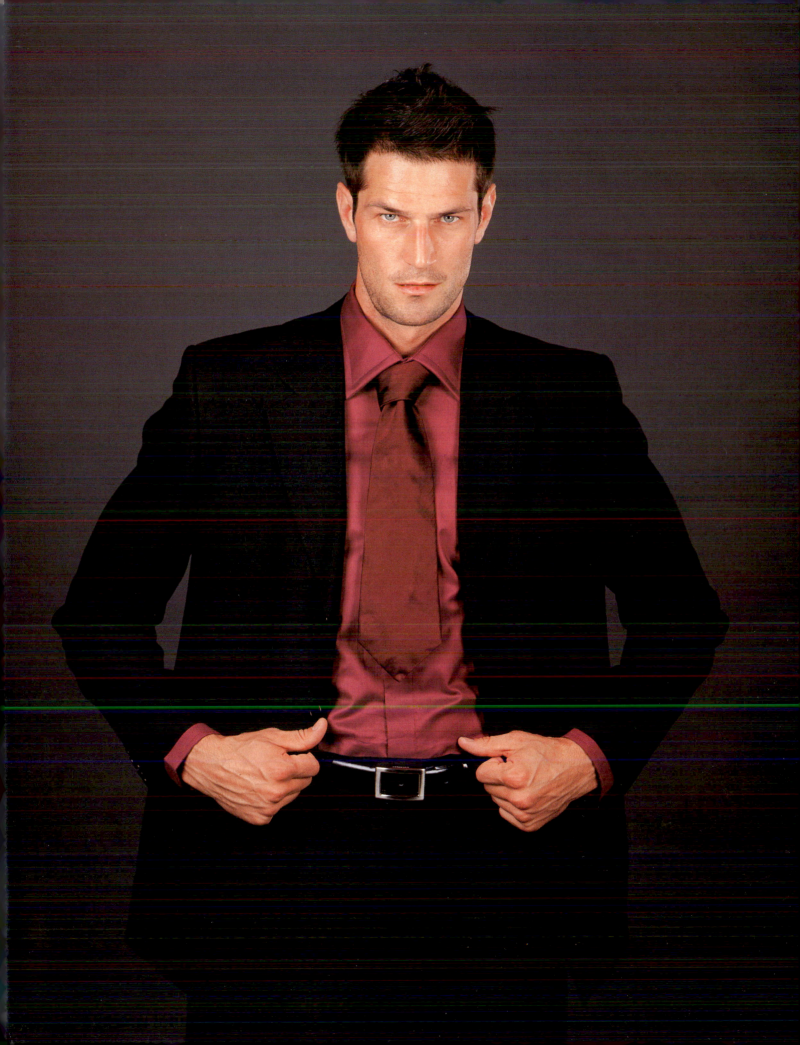

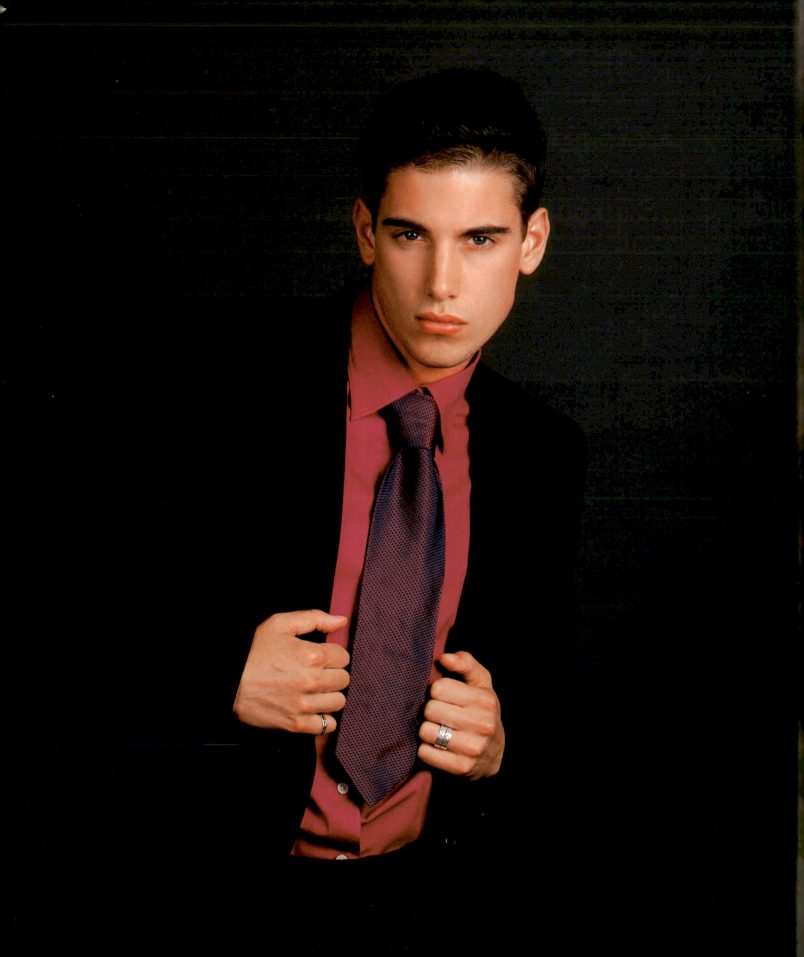

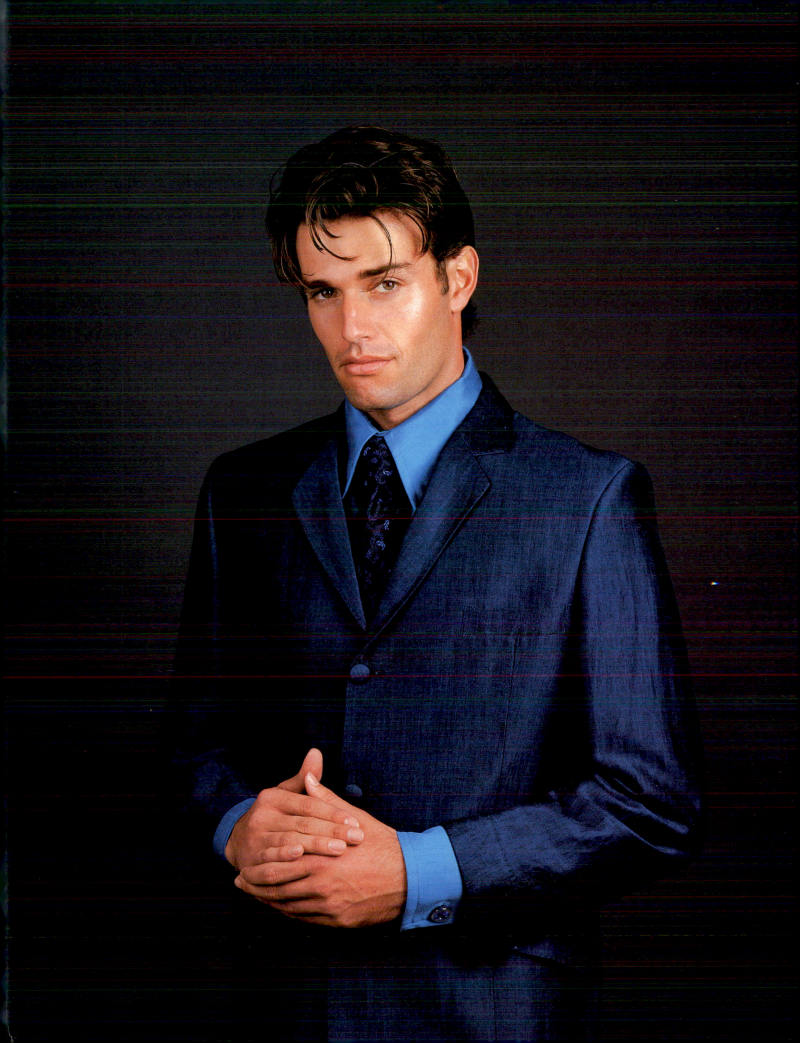

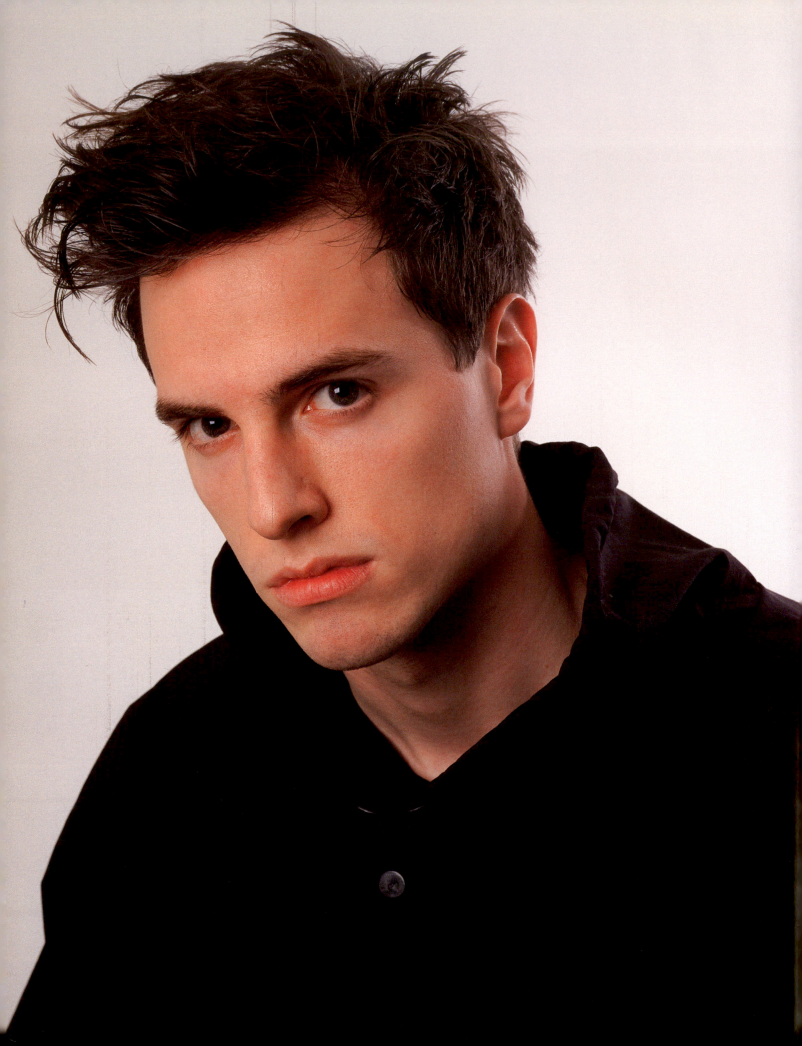

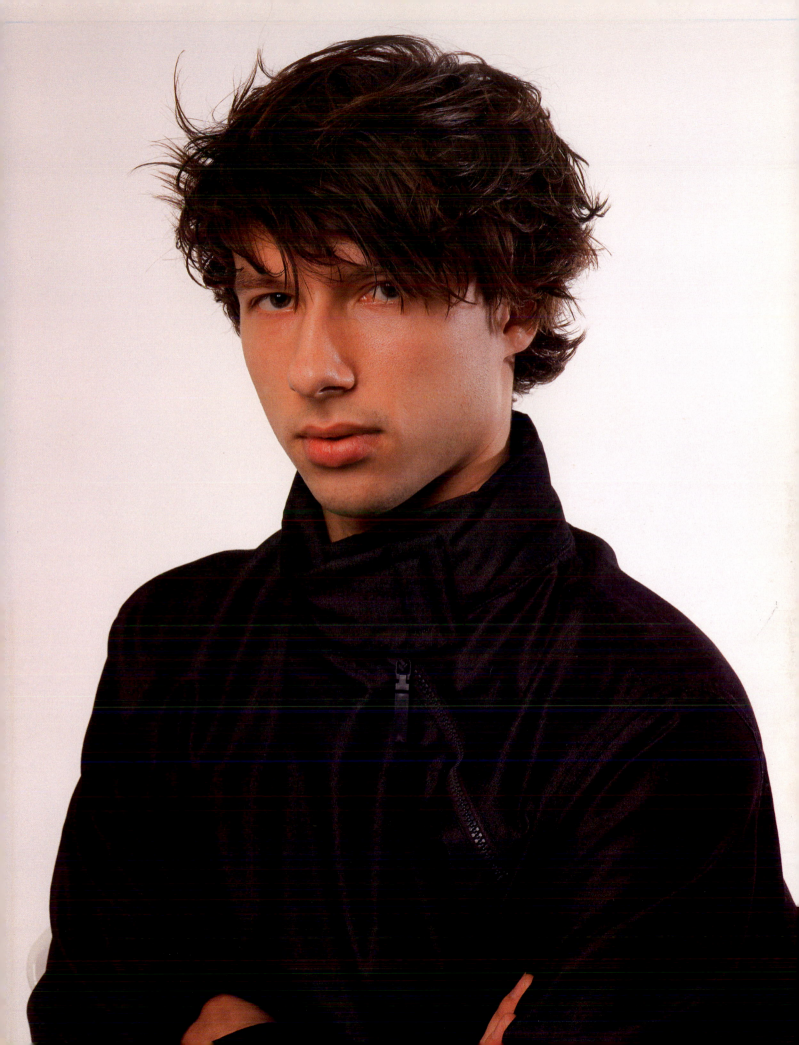

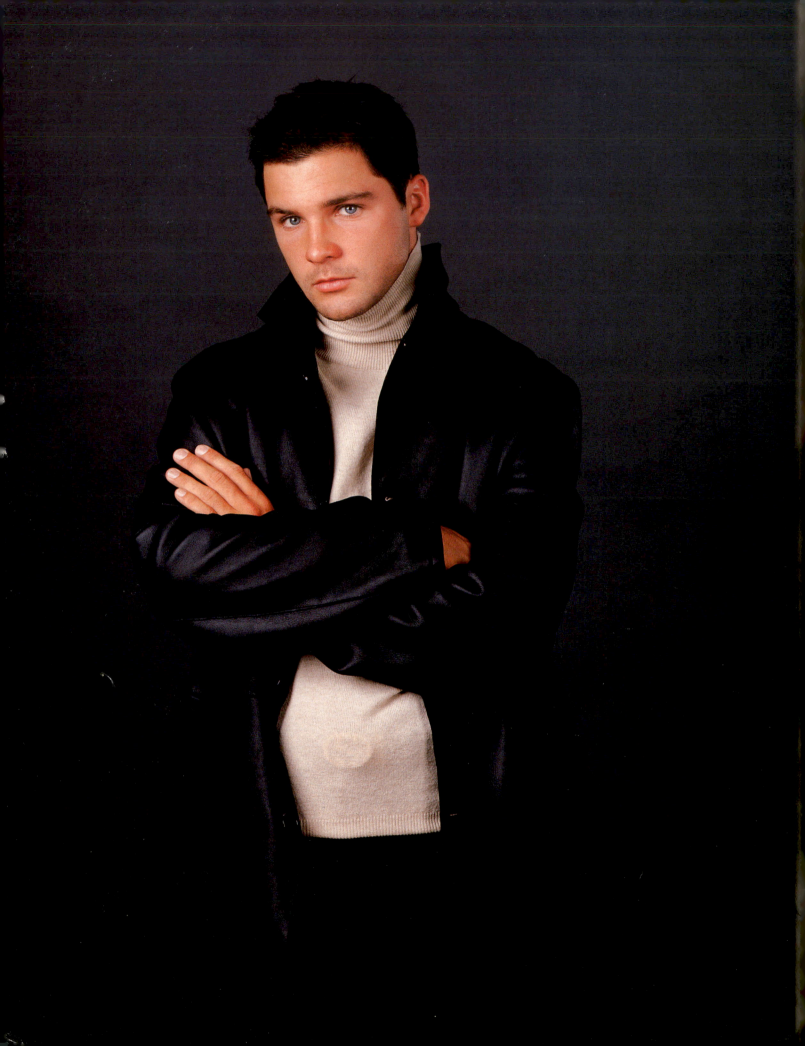

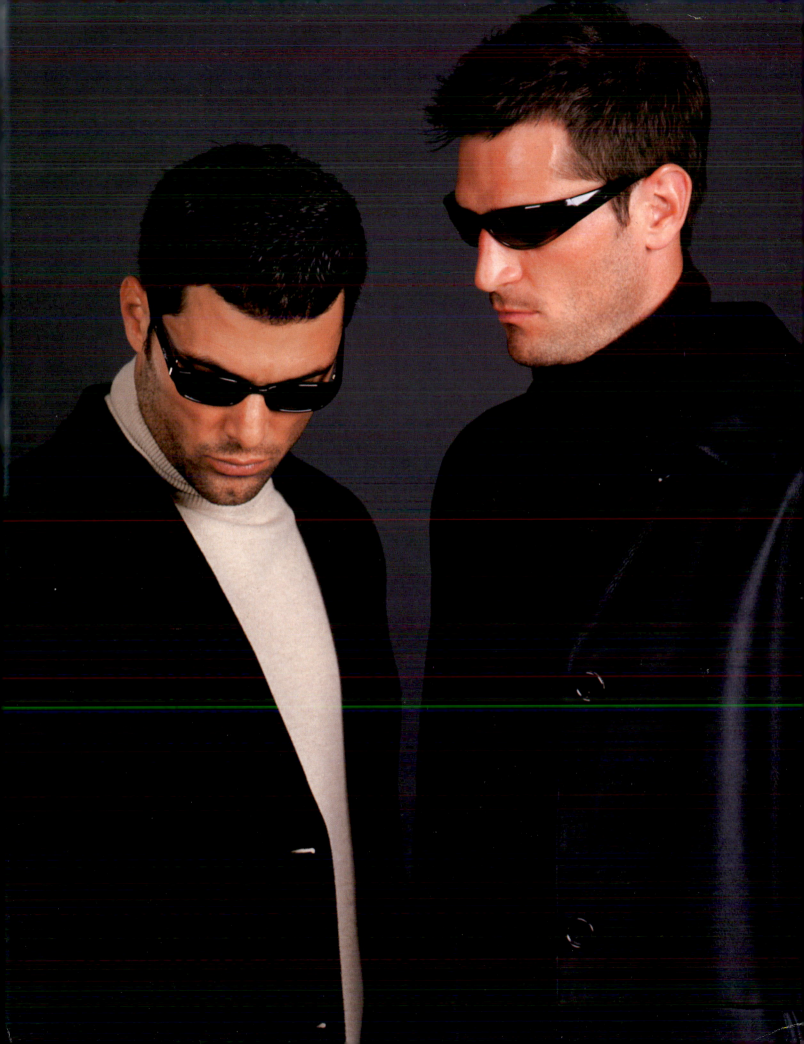

Hairdressing And Beauty Industry Authority series – related titles

HAIRDRESSING

Mahogany Hairdressing: Steps to Cutting, Colouring and Finishing Hair by Martin Gannon and Richard Thompson

Mahogany Hairdressing: Advanced Looks by Richard Thompson and Martin Gannon

Essensuals, Next Generation Toni & Guy Step by Step

Patrick Cameron: Dressing Long Hair by Patrick Cameron and Jacki Wadeson

Patrick Cameron: Dressing Long Hair Book 2 by Patrick Cameron

Bridal Hair by Pat Dixon and Jacki Wadeson

Trevor Sorbie: Visions in Hair by Kris Sorbie and Jacki Wadeson

The Total Look: The Style Guide for Hair and Make-Up Professionals by Ian Mistlin

Art of Hair Colouring by David Adams and Jacki Wadeson

Start Hairdressing: The Official Guide to Level 1 by Martin Green and Leo Palladino

Hairdressing – The Foundations: The Official Guide to Level 2 by Leo Palladino

Professional Hairdressing: The Official Guide to Level 3 by Martin Green, Lesley Kimber and Leo Palladino

Men's Hairdressing: Traditional and Modern Barbering by Maurice Lister

African-Caribbean Hairdressing, 2e by Sandra Gittens

The World of Hair: A Scientific Companion by Dr John Gray

Salon Management by Martin Green

BEAUTY THERAPY

Beauty Therapy – The Foundations: The Official Guide to Level 2 by Lorraine Nordmann

Professional Beauty Therapy: The Official Guide to Level 3 by Lorraine Nordmann, Lorraine Appleyard and Pamela Linforth

Aromatherapy for the Beauty Therapist by Valerie Ann Worwood

Indian Head Massage by Muriel Burnham-Airey and Adele O'Keefe

The Official Guide to Body Massage by Adele O'Keefe

An Holistic Guide to Anatomy & Physiology by Tina Parsons

The Encyclopedia of Nails by Jacqui Jefford and Anne Swain

The Complete Nail Technician by Marian Newman

The World of Skin Care: A Scientific Companion by Dr John Gray

Safety in the Salon by Elaine Almond